Duffield's Exercise in Water

Third edition

EDITED BY

A. T. SKINNER, MCSP, HT, DipTP
Senior Teacher, The School of Physiotherapy,
The Middlesex Hospital, London

and

A. M. THOMSON, MCSP, DipTP
Deputy Principal, The School of Physiotherapy,
The Middlesex Hospital, London

BAILLIERE TINDALL
London Philadelphia Toronto
Sydney Tokyo

Baillière Tindall	24–28 Oval Road
W.B. Saunders	London NW1 7DX

The Curtis Center
Independence Square West
Philadelphia, PA 19106-3399, USA

1 Goldthorne Avenue
Toronto, Ontario M8Z 5T9, Canada

Harcourt Brace Jovanovich (Australia) Pty Ltd
32–52 Smidmore Street, Marrickville
NSW 2204, Australia

Harcourt Brace Jovanovich (Japan) Inc.
Ichibancho Central Building, 22-1 Ichibancho
Chiyoda-ku, Tokyo 102, Japan

First published 1969
Second Edition 1976
Third Edition 1983
 Reprinted 1986 and 1989

Phototypeset by Wyvern Typesetting Ltd, Bristol
Printed and bound in Great Britain by
The Alden Press, Oxford

British Library Cataloguing in Publication Data
Duffield's exercise in water.—3rd ed.
 1. Hydrotherapy
 I. Duffield, M. H.   II. Skinner, A. T.
 III. Thomson, A. M.
 615.8′53 RM811

ISBN 0-7020-0925-3

Contributors

Mrs M. J. Campion (formerly Mrs M. J. Reid) MCSP, MAPA,
Lecturer in Physiotherapy, Western Australia Institute of Technology. Formerly Deputy Superintendent Physiotherapist, Great Ormond Street Hospital for Sick Children, London; and Superintendent Physiotherapist, The Franklin Delano Roosevelt School for Physically Handicapped Children, London

Mrs D. Magonet, SRP,
Formerly Senior Physiotherapist, Hydrotherapy Unit, The Middlesex Hospital, London

Miss A. T. Skinner, MCSP, HT, DipTP,
Senior Teacher, The School of Physiotherapy, The Middlesex Hospital, London

Miss A. M. Thomson, MCSP, DipTP,
Deputy Principal, The School of Physiotherapy, The Middlesex Hospital, London

This book is dedicated to Mary Ainsworth
who did so much to encourage and inspire others
to further their knowledge of hydrotherapy

Contents

Foreword

The third edition of *Duffield's Exercise in Water* has been edited jointly by Miss Alison Skinner and Miss Ann Thomson, both of whom are members of the teaching staff of the Middlesex Hospital School of Physiotherapy. They were both contributors to the earlier editions of this book.

As a teacher of hydrotherapy Miss Skinner is fully conversant with the theory and practice of hydrotherapy and with the problems that confront many students.

Miss Thomson's considerable experience in the treatment of patients will contribute greatly to those chapters concerning the clinical aspects of this subject.

I am sure that this revised edition will prove to be of great assistance to both qualified physiotherapists and to students in training.

M. H. Duffield.

Preface

Following the publication of the Second Edition Miss Duffield asked us to undertake the editing of any future editions and we are pleased to do so. Since 1965 pool therapy has been included in the curriculum to be followed by students studying for the membership examination of the Chartered Society of Physiotherapy. This edition, as with previous editions, is intended for the use of physiotherapy students, clinical physiotherapists who are working in hydrotherapy departments and teachers who wish to learn the basic principles and update their knowledge.

All the chapters have been reviewed. The order of the initial chapters has been altered and some chapters have been renamed. We have included the design and equipment of a hydrotherapy department in Chapter 2. The 'principles of treatment' chapters have now been divided into a chapter on general procedures, including the progression of exercises, followed by a chapter on specialized techniques including those developed at Bad Ragaz in Switzerland. These techniques have been greatly expanded and include line diagrams which we hope will make the techniques easier to follow. Miss Bridget Davis, District Physiotherapist, Camberwell Health Authority, introduced these techniques to this country and we are indebted to her. This chapter also includes repeated contractions, rhythmic stabilizations and breathing exercises adapted for the pool.

The chapter on the Halliwick method has been expanded by Mrs M. Campion (formerly Reid) to include the treatment of adults. This chapter owes much to the President Emeritus of the Association of Swimming Therapy, Mr J. McMillan, MBE, for his advice and experience. The chapters on conditions commonly treated in the pool have been revised to bring them into line with present trends, and references have been made to chapters on the principles of treatment where appropriate. We hope the applications of the theoretical chapters is thereby more evident. We have continued to include lists of exercises as examples for those with little experience and hope these will provide a basis for a varied treatment programme. The terminology has been standardized and used throughout so that the exercises can be understood. A section on Health and Safety has been included.

There are a number of new photographs particularly related to the treatment of patients and for these we wish to thank the members of staff of the photographic department of the Middlesex Hospital for their help and patience in taking them. The photograph in Fig. 2.2 is reproduced by kind permission of Mr Peter Wells, Superintendent Physiotherapist, and Mr Lyons, House Governor, both of St Stephen's Hospital, London.

We are grateful to a number of people who have helped and encouraged us with the preparation of this edition. We thank Mrs D Magonet and Mrs M. Campion (formerly Reid) for their contribution to the chapters on conditions; Mrs C. Mabey for her understanding and cooperation in the experiments carried out in the hydrotherapy department; Miss Mary Archer, who spent many hours typing and re-typing our efforts; Mr Smith and the staff at Baillière Tindall for their patience and assistance, and the Physiotherapy Staff at the Middlesex Hospital for their comments and encouragement.

December 1982   A. T. Skinner
                                                     A. M. Thomson

Introduction

The term hydrotherapy is derived from the Greek words *hydor*—water, and *therapeia*—healing. There is no very clear evidence as to when water was first used for healing purposes but it is known that Hippocrates (*c*. 460–375 BC) used hot and cold water (contrast baths) in the treatment of disease. Water for recreational and curative purposes was used widely by the Romans. They had four types of bath of varying temperature: the frigidarium was a cold bath and was used only for recreational purposes; the tepidarium consisted of a tepid bath sited in a room containing warm air; the caldarium contained a hot bath and the sudatorium was a room filled with moist hot air to promote sweating. The remains of these baths may still be seen at Bath and Buxton and many other places both in this country and abroad.

Little more was heard of this method of treatment until 1697 when Sir John Flayer, a physician living in Lichfield, published a paper on 'An Enquiry into the Right Use and Abuse of Hot, Cold and Temperate Baths in England'. He followed this 25 years later with a 'History of Cold Bathing'. He advocated that hot baths should be used in hot countries and cold baths in cold countries, but he himself opened a centre for tepid baths in Lichfield. In spite of dedicating his second paper to the Royal College of Physicians his teaching received little support in England, although in Germany tepid baths were used extensively for the relief of muscle spasm and in the treatment of hyper-excitable patients.

In 1779 a ship's surgeon, Doctor Wright, published his findings on the use of cold in the treatment of smallpox, and subsequently he used this form of treatment for many febrile conditions at a clinic he opened in Edinburgh. He stimulated Doctor Currie, a Liverpool physician, to investigate further the effects produced by cold, and he published a paper on 'Medical Reports of the Effect of Water, Cold and Warm, as a Remedy for Fever'. He advocated the 'subtraction of heat' for sedation of the nervous system. Although

Currie's methods were used widely on the Continent, they did not find favour with the medical profession in England.

In 1830 a Silesian peasant, Vincent Pressnitz, set up a centre for the use of cold water and vigorous exercise. These methods did receive some support in this country, but centres which were opened in Matlock and Malvern did not survive for long as they were used chiefly by unqualified practitioners and were looked down on by the medical profession. However, Pressnitz stimulated considerable thought on the Continent and for the first time scientific investigation was undertaken into the reactions of the tissues to water at various temperatures, and their reaction in disease. Taking part in these investigations was Doctor Winterwitz of Vienna, who made a further study of the works of Wright and Currie, finally establishing an accepted physiological basis for hydrotherapy.

As in this country, there was considerable opposition at first to the therapeutic use of water in France, Italy and America, but gradually it gained favour in these countries and treatment centres were established in all of them, although it was not until 1903 that the first centre was opened in the United States, in Boston.

Like many other forms of treatment, the use of hydrotherapy met with suspicion at first, partly because unsupported and extravagant claims were made for its effects and value. Gradually, however, it became accepted as a recognized form of treatment for nervous and other disorders. It is interesting to note that early emphasis was laid on the use of cold, and today ice has become an increasingly popular form of treatment for, among other conditions, the relief of muscle spasm.

At the beginning of this century treatment in the spas in this country was given by people with little training or medical knowledge and it was available only to those members of the community who could afford to visit them. The many physicians who specialized in the treatment of rheumatism felt that this was unsatisfactory, and largely at their instigation the British Red Cross Society opened a clinic for the treatment of Rheumatic Diseases at Peto Place in London. It was formally opened by Her Majesty Queen Mary in 1930 and it was staffed by chartered physiotherapists with Miss McAllister, SRN, CSMMG, in charge. The Council of the Chartered Society then approved a syllabus for a post-registration training in hydrotherapy to be taken at this clinic. This was quickly superseded by a longer 12-week course followed by an examination. Soon after this, a similar training course was started in Cardiff and later in Bath, Buxton and Harrogate. With some modifications this training has continued to the present day, but recently it was decided that the principles of pool therapy should be included in the 3-year course for physiotherapists and the post-registration courses as such have ceased to exist.

1

Basic Physical Principles and Their Application

In order to understand the principles of hydrotherapy it is necessary to acquire a knowledge of the physical properties of water, particularly in their relation to the concepts of matter.

Matter. Anything that occupies space is known as matter. It is composed of molecules which, in turn, are composed of atoms. All matter exists in three forms: as solids, liquids or gases. Water is an example of a substance which can exist in any of the three states—ice, water and steam. Below 0°C (32°F) water is solid, between 0°C (32°F) and 100°C (212°F) it is liquid, and above 100°C (212°F), gaseous.

PHYSICAL PROPERTIES OF WATER

In common with other forms of matter, water has certain physical properties which include: mass, weight, density, specific gravity, buoyancy, hydrostatic pressure, surface tension, refraction and viscosity.

MASS
The mass of a substance is the amount of material it comprises.

WEIGHT
The weight of a substance is the force with which it is attracted towards the centre of the earth.

Relationship between mass and weight. Mass is unalterable and is measured in pounds or kilograms. Weight is the effect of gravity upon the mass, and alters according to the position of a body in relation to the earth. Units of measurement are newtons (N) in the MKS system (Système Internationale d'Unités, SI system). This system has now replaced the FPS and CGS systems. A newton is the force which, acting on a mass of 1 kg for 1 s, generates a velocity of 1 m/s.

$$W = Ma$$

where W = weight, M = mass and a = acceleration due to gravity. The force of gravity is approximately 9·81 m/s^2.
A mass of 1 kg has a weight of 9·81 N.

DENSITY
A wooden log weighing 100 kg will float but an iron nail weighing a few grams will sink; this is because wood is less dense than iron.
The density of a substance is the relationship between its mass and its volume:

$$\text{density} = \frac{\text{mass}}{\text{volume}}$$

Mass per unit volume is expressed as grams per cubic centimetre (g/cm^3) or kilograms per cubic metre (kg/m^3). Water is most dense at 4°C (39·2°F). It expands at both higher and lower temperatures and therefore ice is less dense than water and floats (Fig. 1.1). The density of ice is 920 kg/m^3, that of iron 7700 kg/m^3, that of wood 750 kg/m^3; the average density of the human body is 950 kg/m^3. Dissolved substances increase the density of water; therefore, sea water for example is denser (1024 kg/m^3) than pure water (1000 kg/m^3).

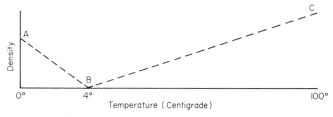

Fig. 1.1. Change in density of water with temperature variation. (Broken line shows the expansion of water.)

RELATIVE DENSITY

The relative density or specific gravity of a substance is the ratio of the mass of a given volume of the substance to the mass of the same volume of water. The relative density of pure water is 1; a body with a specific gravity of less than 1 will float, and a body with more than 1 will sink in water.

BUOYANCY

Of the physical laws of water that the hydrotherapist should understand and apply when giving pool therapy, those of buoyancy (Archimedes' principle), and of hydrostatic pressure (Pascal's law) are most important.

Archimedes' principle. The principle of Archimedes states that when a body is wholly or partially immersed in a fluid at rest it experiences an upthrust equal to the weight of fluid displaced. Therefore, if a body has a relative density of less than 1 it will float, since the weight of the object is less than the weight of water displaced. If the relative density is greater than 1 it will sink, and if equal to 1 it will float just below the surface of the water.

Since the relative density of the human body with air in the lungs is 0·95, it will float. When the body is floating the ratio of the submerged parts to those which are not submerged is 0·95:0·05. If the unsubmerged portion of the body exceeds 0·05, as when a person has the head and arms fixed above the water level, the amount of water displaced by the remainder will be insufficient to support the weight of the body and the pelvis and legs will sink. However, placing a float round the pelvis reduces the relative density of the lower part of the body, which will then not sink (Figs 1.2–1.4).

A submarine can submerge or float at will because its density can be altered by increasing or decreasing the proportion of air to water in the ballast tanks. Similarly, in the human body, the density can be altered by increasing or decreasing the amount of air in the lungs.

Fig. 1.2. Body floating at rest.

Buoyancy - the tendency of to rise or float in a fluid, Results from the upward thrust equal to weight of fluid of displaced

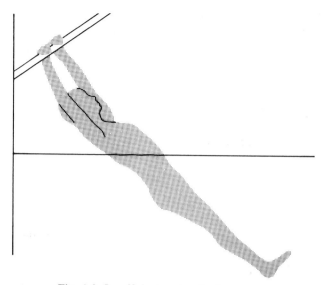

Fig. 1.3. Insufficient water displacement.

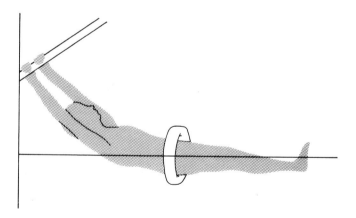

Fig. 1.4. Use of pelvic float.

Hence a person whose lungs are filled with air on inspiration will float, but he will sink when he breathes out on expiration.

As wood has a specific gravity of less than 1, wooden sticks or crutches used in the pool must be made more dense than water by adding weights at their ends; alternatively, they can be made of solid metal. The amount of support or resistance given to a patient by inflatable floats can be varied by increasing or decreasing the amount of air in them, thereby altering their density.

Buoyancy is the force experienced as an upthrust which acts in the opposite direction to the force of gravity. A body in water is therefore subjected to two opposing forces—gravity, acting through the centre of gravity, and buoyancy, acting through the centre of buoyancy which is the centre of gravity of the displaced liquid. When the weight of the floating body equals the weight of the liquid displaced, and the centres of buoyancy and gravity are in the same vertical line, the body is kept in stable equilibrium. If the centres are not in the same vertical line the two forces acting on the body will cause it to roll over until it reaches a position of stable equilibrium (Figs 1.5 and 1.6).

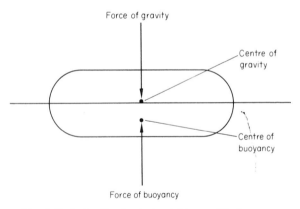

Force of gravity

Centre of gravity

Centre of buoyancy

Force of buoyancy

Fig. 1.5. A floating body in stable equilibrium.

Moment of force. The moment of force about a point is the turning effect of the force about that point. As buoyancy is itself a force, this rule will govern its action.

Moment of buoyancy. This is represented by

$$F \times d$$

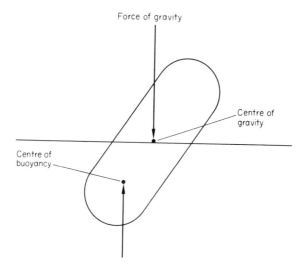

Fig. 1.6. Interaction of gravity and buoyancy.

where F = the force of buoyancy, d = the perpendicular distance from a vertical line through X to the centre of buoyancy, and X = the point about which the turning effect of buoyancy is exerted.

Figure 1.7 illustrates this principle by showing the force of buoyancy and the centre of buoyancy on a lever submerged in water at three different angles. The moment of buoyancy on

$$AB_1 = F \times d_1$$

and on

$$AB_2 = F \times d_2$$

As d_2 is greater than d_1 the moment of force is greater on AB_2 than on AB_1. In the vertical position d = zero, so there is no turning effect, but as the level comes to the surface the effect is increased and is maximal at B_3 where d_3 is greatest.

In the human body the lever is formed by the limbs, X being the joint about which movement is occurring. When X represents the shoulder joint, and the upper limb is AB, the moment of force, i.e. the turning effect of buoyancy, increases with the degree of abduction. The effect of buoyancy therefore increases as the limb approaches the surface of the water (Fig. 1.8). If the lever is shortened by bending the elbow, the centre of buoyancy moves nearer to X, the distance d is shortened and the moment of

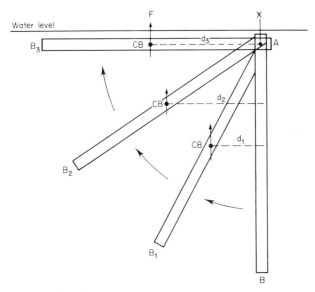

Fig. 1.7. The turning effect of buoyancy. A lever (A-B) is submerged in water. F = force of buoyancy; CB = centre of buoyancy; d = distance from vertical; X = point about which turning effect is exerted.

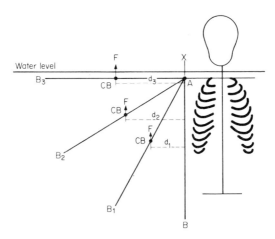

Fig. 1.8. Effect of buoyancy increasing on abduction. Key as for Fig. 1.7.

buoyancy is less (Fig. 1.9). Buoyancy, therefore, will have a greater effect on a long rather than a short lever.

Buoyancy may be used to assist a movement when the limb is moved towards the surface of the water, and to resist movement when the limb is moved from the surface of the water to the vertical position. The moment of buoyancy increases (a) as the limb moves nearer to the surface of the water, and (b) as the lever lengthens. Therefore, when strengthening weak muscles, a longer lever and movement nearer the horizontal gain the most assistance from buoyancy. However, when the movement is carried out against the force of buoyancy, there will be resistance to the movement which lessens (a) as the limb nears the vertical position, and (b) with a shorter lever. The maximum resistance of buoyancy is thus exerted on a long lever near to the horizontal.

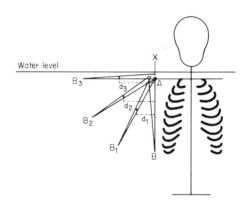

Fig. 1.9. A weaker effect due to bending the elbow. Key as for Fig. 1.7.

The assistance or resistance of buoyancy can be increased still further by using floats which alter the position of the centre of buoyancy, and so the distance between the centre and the point about which the force of buoyancy exerts its turning effect. In Fig. 1.10(a), d_{1-3} is shorter than in Fig. 1.10(b), and so the moment of force has increased.

When a person stands almost upright in water his body tends to return to the vertical position, but during walking or sitting the legs tend to be displaced to the surface if they are raised too high and the

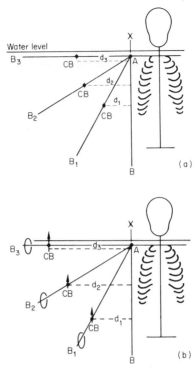

Fig. 1.10. Effect of buoyancy altered by addition of float. Key as for Fig. 1.7.

body overbalances backwards (Figs 1.11 and 1.12). The 'weight relief' of the body due to the upthrust of buoyancy is one of the main advantages of pool treatment.

HYDROSTATIC PRESSURE

The molecules of a fluid exert a thrust upon each part of the surface area of an immersed body. This thrust per unit area is the pressure of the fluid. Pascal's law states that fluid pressure is exerted equally on all surface areas of an immersed body at rest at a given depth (Fig. 1.13(a)). Pressure increases (a) with the density of the fluid, and (b) with its depth. For example, the pressure exerted by alcohol is less than that of water and the pressure exerted by sea water is more than that of pure water at a given depth.

The pressure of the water is felt when a person enters the pool. It

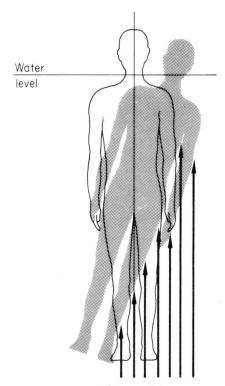

Water
level

Force of buoyancy

Fig. 1.11. Temporary displacement of vertical body.

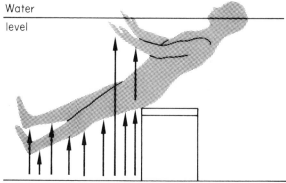

Water
level

Force of buoyancy

Fig. 1.12. Displacement during activity.

is most evident on the chest, where the water resists expansion (Fig. 1.13(b)), so it is usually advisable to assess patients with a vital capacity of less than 1000 cm³ before allowing them into a pool. Owing to the pressure of the water, which may be 488·24 kg/m², care should be taken when treating weak patients. Being equal in all directions, the pressure is not felt more on one surface of the body than another, and will give uniform resistance at a given depth. Since pressure increases with depth, swelling will be reduced more easily if exercises are given well below the surface of the water where the increased pressure may be used. The lateral pressure exerted and the effect of buoyancy together will give the feeling of weightlessness.

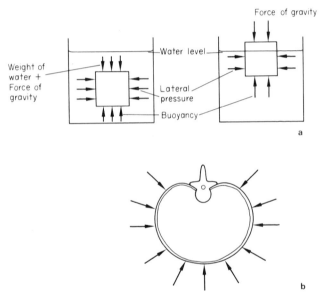

Fig. 1.13. (a) Pressure on a floating body; (b) pressure on all aspects of the thorax, opposing expansion.

Cohesion and adhesion. Cohesion is the force of attraction between neighbouring molecules of the same type of matter. Adhesion is the force of attraction between neighbouring molecules of different types of matter.

When water is placed in a container there is, therefore, a cohesive force between the molecules of the water and an adhesive force between the water and both the container and the molecules of the air above. The cohesive force of the water molecules themselves and the adhesive force between the molecules of the water and the container are greater than the adhesive force between the water and the air above (Fig. 1.14). In this way, the upper surface molecules are drawn downwards and the surface of the water in the container is concave. The adhesive force between the container and the water molecules is greater than the cohesive force of the water, and this results in the walls of the container remaining wet after the water is removed.

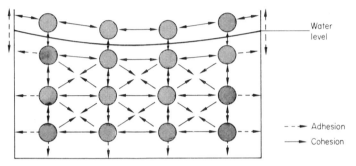

Fig. 1.14. Cohesive and adhesive forces.

SURFACE TENSION

This is the force exerted between the surface molecules of a fluid. The force is probably due to cohesion between the molecules and manifests itself as an elastic 'skin' at the surface of the fluid. The tendency is thus for the area at the surface to try to contract to a minimum. The surface tension of water can be demonstrated by floating a needle on the surface of the water.

Surface tension acts as a resistance to movement when a limb is partially submerged as the surface tension has to be broken by the movement, but the effect is slight and is of value only if the muscles are small or weak.

REFRACTION

This is the bending of a ray as it passes from a more to a less dense medium or vice versa. When a ray passes from a rarer to a denser medium, as from air to water, it bends towards the normal; passage in the opposite direction, from a denser to a rarer medium, bends the ray away from the normal. The normal is an imaginary line drawn at right angles to the interface of the two media at the point where the ray strikes. (Figs 1.15 and 1.16).

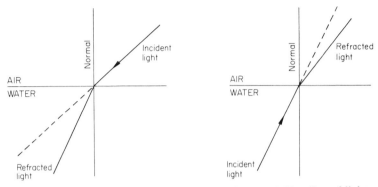

Fig. 1.15. Bending of light towards the normal.

Fig. 1.16. Bending of light away from the normal.

Let us consider a ray of light reflected from the bottom of the pool (Fig. 1.17). The ray will be refracted away from the normal as it passes from the water to the air; hence point A appears to occur at point B because the observer assumes that light travels in a straight line. The pool, therefore, seems to be shallower than it is. The patient's limbs appear distorted, those partially submerged seeming to be bent away from the normal at water level. This means that movement of joints may be difficult to observe.

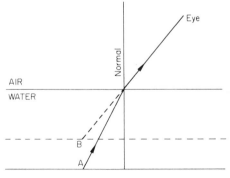

Fig. 1.17. The effect of refraction on light rays reflected from the bottom of the pool.
A = true bottom; B = false bottom.

VISCOSITY

This is the type of friction that occurs between the molecules of a liquid and causes a resistance to flow of the liquid. Such friction expresses the viscosity—the 'stickiness' or the ease with which the liquid flows—and therefore is only noticeable when the fluid is in motion. Any liquid with a high viscosity, such as thick oil, flows slowly, and those with a low viscosity such as water will flow more quickly and offer less resistance.

Viscosity acts as a resistance to movement as the molecules of a liquid tend to adhere to the surface of a body moving through it. When an object moves through a fluid of high viscosity there is greater turbulence at a given speed and therefore greater resistance to the movement. If the temperature of the liquid is raised, however, its viscosity is reduced because the molecules are further apart.

The viscosity of blood is greater than that of water and depends on its contents. This is a factor influencing blood pressure. Air is less viscid than water; therefore there is more resistance to movement in the pool than on the land. The viscosity of the warm water in the pool is less than in cold sea water.

Movement through water

The behaviour of a fluid is controlled by the nature and rate of flow. Professor Osborne Reynolds (1849–1912) demonstrated that the flow of a liquid may be either streamlined or turbulent. He injected dye at constant velocity into a stream of fluid and found that when the fluid flowed slowly the dye appeared as a thread in the stream (streamline or laminar flow), but when the flow was increased the dye twisted and eventually mixed completely with the fluid (turbulent flow). Turbulent flow is produced when the velocity of flow is increased beyond a certain level—the *critical velocity*. Liquids of a high viscosity have a high critical velocity.

Streamline flow is a continuous steady movement of fluid, the rate of movement at any fixed point remaining constant. It can be pictured as very thin layers of fluid molecules sliding over one another, the inner layers moving quickly, the outer ones moving slowly, and the outermost ones remaining stationary (Fig. 1.18).

Turbulent flow is an irregular movement of the fluid, the movement varying at any fixed point (Fig. 1.19). This type of flow creates occasional rotary movements called eddies. It can be visualized as rapid, random movements of fluid molecules.

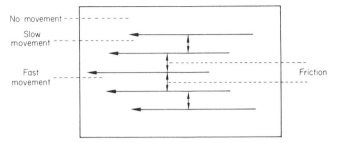

Fig. 1.18. Streamline flow.

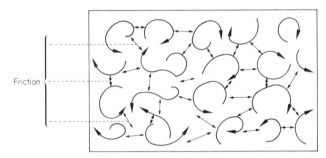

Fig. 1.19. Turbulent flow.

Frictional resistance due to turbulent flow is greater than that due to streamline flow. In streamline flow resistance is directly proportional to velocity, while in turbulent flow resistance is proportional to the square of the velocity. The resistance offered by streamline flow is due to friction between layers of the fluid molecules only, whereas in turbulent flow the resistance is due to friction both between individual fluid molecules (as opposed to layers), and between the fluid and the container surface.

When an object moves through water, a difference in water pressure develops between the front and the back of the object. The pressure builds up in front and decreases at the rear, resulting in a flow of water into the area of reduced pressure—known as 'the wake' (Fig. 1.20). Eddies form in the wake, partly from the water round the edges, and partly from the water behind the object. Flow in the wake is thus impeded, tending to drag the object back. The faster the movement, the greater is the drag, and therefore the greater the resistance to movement. If the movement is suddenly

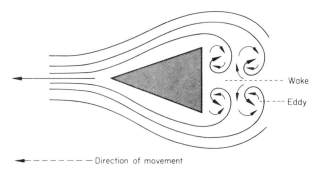

Fig. 1.20. Formation of wake and eddies.

reversed, it is opposed by the inertia of the water, and turbulence occurs. Similarly, if the wake hits the side of the container the rebound causes turbulence.

Streamlined and unstreamlined bodies. When a broad-ended object moves through water the streamlines (imaginary lines in the fluid) break away from the surface of the object and form waves which travel sideways away from it, becoming gradually weaker. The object is said to be 'unstreamlined' (Fig. 1.21). With a narrow object moving through water there is little or no breakaway of the

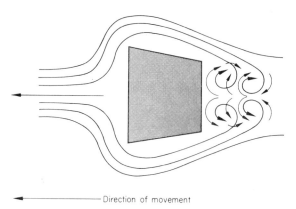

Fig. 1.21. Unstreamlined object.

streamlines, and little disturbance of the water (Fig. 1.22)—the object is said to be 'streamlined'. With an unstreamlined body there is greater wave formation and so greater resistance to its movement.

Streamline refers to the shape of a body in which imaginary lines are to travel near normal object a little breakaway. A streamlined body causes few waves and needs little to do normmay

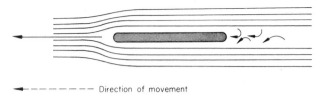

Direction of movement

Fig. 1.22. Streamlined object.

Practical applications of turbulence

1. Turbulence can be used as a form of resistance to exercises in the pool. The quicker the movement, the greater the turbulence, and therefore an exercise may be progressed by increasing the speed at which it is taken.

2. Floats and bats can be made streamlined or unstreamlined, thus altering the resistance to movement: the narrow surface moving against the water offers little resistance but the flat surface offers maximum resistance to the water (Figs 1.23 and 1.24). An exercise may therefore be made more difficult by changing from a streamlined to an unstreamlined body.

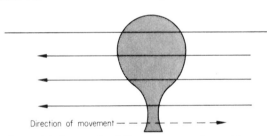

Direction of movement

Fig. 1.23. Streamlined flow across surface of bat.

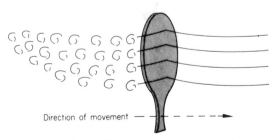

Direction of movement

Fig. 1.24. Bat facing flow of water causing turbulence.

The wake is an area of reduced pressure in the water behind a moving object. If another object is placed in the wake it will move very easily through the water. It is much easier to walk behind another person in his wake than in front of him. Thus when re-educating a patient to walk in the pool a physiotherapist should always walk in front of the patient at first to make it easier for him.

3. Swimming in water is easier than walking because the body is more streamlined when swimming.

HEAT

Heat is a form of energy and when other forms of energy are converted into heat there is a constant ratio between the heat produced and the energy lost. Heat, therefore, can be measured in energy units, and since 1948 the joule (J) has replaced the calorie as the unit of heat.

A calorie is the amount of heat required to raise the temperature of one gram of water from 15°C to 16°C. One calorie = 4·2 J, approximately.

Heat capacity
The amount of heat required to raise the temperature of a body by 1 degree is called its thermal capacity and is measured in joules per degree. It depends on the mass and the substance of the body.

Latent heat
This is the amount of heat, in joules, required to change the state of 1 gram of a substance without raising its temperature. It is, therefore, the energy that is used in changing a solid to a liquid or a liquid to a gas. An equal amount of energy is released when the reverse processes take place.

The conversion of a liquid into a vapour is known as evaporation. It depends on the nature of the fluid, its temperature and that of the atmosphere, the extent of surface area exposed to the air, the degree of saturation of the surrounding air and the amount of air movement.

Evaporation of sweat is one of the most important ways in which the body loses heat after immersion in the pool. The body loses 0·6 calories (about 2·5 J) for every gram of sweat vapourized.

Newton's law of cooling

The rate of cooling of a body in a given time is proportional to the difference in temperature between the body and its surroundings. The greater the difference in temperature the greater will be the rate of cooling. In order to prevent too rapid cooling on leaving the pool, the patient may be wrapped in a warm sheet and blankets and the temperature of the rest room be maintained at 21°C (70°F). To prevent too rapid cooling of the exposed parts of the body during treatment the temperature of the treatment room is maintained at 25°C (80°F).

Humidity. Evaporation is constantly taking place from the surfaces of rivers, wet streets and wet ground, and therefore the air always contains some moisture. The wetness of the air is known as humidity.

Relative humidity is the ratio of the amount of water vapour present in the air to the amount which would be present if the air were saturated at the same temperature. It is usually expressed as a percentage.

Air is able to absorb different amounts of moisture at different temperatures. The higher the temperature, the greater the amount of water vapour that can be absorbed; dry air raises the temperature, damp air lowers it.

The evaporation of sweat produces a cooling of the body. If the air surrounding the body is already fully saturated with water vapour no evaporation can take place and the body cannot lose heat in this way. If the atmospheric temperature is high the body cannot lose heat by conduction, convection or radiation. Therefore, when the humidity and the temperature are both high the body has difficulty in losing heat and conditions become very uncomfortable. In the hydrotherapy department the temperature should be maintained at 20–21°C (68–70°F) and the ideal humidity is 55%. Therefore, proper temperature control and ventilation are essential for the comfort of both patients and staff.

2

Hydrotherapy Department Design and Equipment

The hydrotherapy department is a self-contained unit, with its own changing, rest and utility rooms, and ample storage space for linen and equipment. It is important to avoid draughts in pool and rest room areas, and to this end, the department should be designed with as few doors as possible. It is advisable to avoid having doors with direct outside access, but where this is unavoidable a small porch may be constructed over the door, which must have sufficient width for the easy passage of wheelchairs and stretchers, as indeed must all the other doors and corridors. There should also be sufficient room to turn stretchers round if necessary, and a place for the temporary parking of stretchers and wheelchairs. The size of the department depends on the demands of each hospital, and the types of patient undergoing treatment.

Refreshment facilities are necessary near to the hydrotherapy department so that after the rest period the patient may have a drink to replenish fluid loss.

POOLS AND TANKS

Pools are built with a reinforced concrete shell, a layer of asphalt and a second layer of reinforced concrete.

Prefabricated fibreglass pools are now available in standard sizes, and these can be enlarged by adding another section. Tiles, mosaic, fibreglass or plastics are used as lining materials; if tiles are used they have a rough finish, or the surface is ridged or studded to ensure that they are slip proof. Mosaic is very satisfactory but expensive; fibreglass as a lining is cheaper but not always satisfactory.

The ideal site for a pool is the basement or ground floor of a building, otherwise the weight of water requires considerable ceiling reinforcement and a limitation in size.

Size of pools. The pool itself should be large enough to allow the patient to progress throughout his full rehabilitation programme, from using the full support of a stretcher to partial support, then on to walking and, ideally, to swimming and other recreational activities.

A pool measuring 2·5 by 3 m can accommodate at most two patients and a physiotherapist at one time but its use is limited. A pool 4 by 6 m can take seven or eight people, who may be equal numbers of patients and physiotherapists or more patients and fewer physiotherapists. Thus the larger the pool, the greater the use to which it can be put. When swimming is an integral part of the patient's rehabilitation, as in the treatment of spinal injuries, a much larger area of, say, 9 by 4·5 m is necessary. According to a survey conducted by K. R. Greenless* on therapy pools in Britain, their sizes vary from 7·43 to 32·54 m², the largest group (32%) having an area 13·94 to 18·58 m².

SUNKEN AND RAISED POOLS

Pools can be either sunken or raised, the former type being constructed at promenade level while the latter is surmounted by an 800-mm wall. The choice is largely a matter of individual preference, but a good case can be made for each type. In a new building there is little difference in the cost of erection, but a raised pool may be a more suitable choice for installation in an existing building. Some engineers believe that the raised pool is easier to maintain and keep clean.

The sunken pool (Fig. 2.1) is surmounted by a kerb about 200 mm high, and has steps by which the patient can enter. These may be built into the pool or made of teak and fixed to one wall. In this type of pool the patient has fewer steps to negotiate than in the

*Available from Arthur F. Houghton & Associates, 14 St Andrews Road, West Town, Backwell, Bristol.

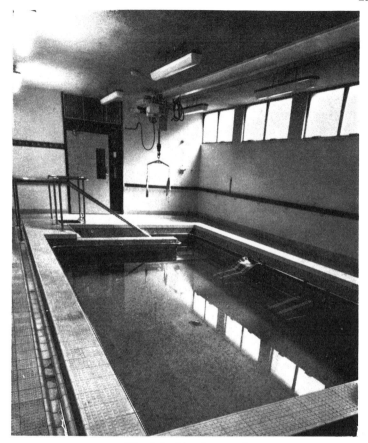

Fig. 2.1. A sunken pool.

raised pool, and since the water level is lower relative to the height of the ceiling, air is able to circulate more freely. Use of a sunken pool makes it necessary for the physiotherapist to be in the pool while treating the patient. Many authorities believe this ensures the best possible treatment; fixation of the patient by the physiotherapist is firmer, and she has more control over his movements.

The raised or free-standing pool has an outer wall 200 mm wide and 800 mm high (Fig. 2.2). It slopes slightly outward towards the foot to a recess at floor level under which the physiotherapist can tuck her feet when she leans over the wall to a patient in the pool

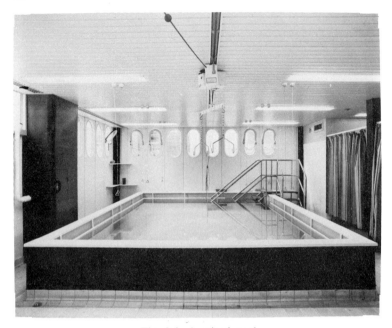

Fig. 2.2. A raised pool.

(Fig. 2.3). The water level should be between 130 mm and 200 mm from the top of the wall.

With this type of pool, communication with the patient is easier; and in a busy department with a small staff, it may also be an advantage to control some patients from outside the pool, thus allowing the physiotherapist to treat more patients than with a sunken pool where her time in the pool itself must be restricted. On the other hand, fixation, and thus control, of the patient is less localized from the side, and the physiotherapist's back is at risk.

All pools, whatever their size or type, should have some method of removing scum.

Pool floor and depth. The floor of the pool may be level, sloping or graded in two or three depths. A level floor allows freedom of range over the whole pool, and a 1·1-m depth of water gives sufficient buoyancy for all patients. In addition, this type of floor allows most adult patients to walk with confidence, and enables even a short physiotherapist to maintain a firm foothold and therefore a good control of the patient during exercise. In some

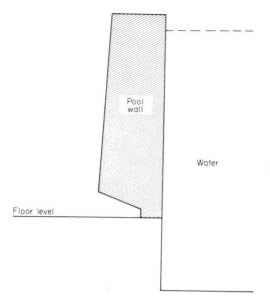

Fig. 2.3. Cross-section of a raised pool.

pools the depth of the water can be altered, though it may take time for the water to reach the correct temperature at the new level.

It is possible to have a pool with a perforated, moveable floor which can be altered in height and this has the effect of altering the depth of the water, as required. This is ideal but very expensive.

The usual *gradient* for a pool with a sloping floor is 1 in 15. A sloping floor can be most satisfactory in a large pool, and where swimming plays an important part both in rehabilitation and recreational activities; all patients will benefit from performing their exercises in the depth of water most suitable to their height.

A *graded floor* usually has three depths of water, stepped lanes running the length of the pool. The demarcation between each step must be made very clearly visible by using tiles of different colours on the edge of each step. The graded pool is particularly useful if both adults and children are being treated. The grading is also an asset in progressing exercises for walking from deep to shallower water, with a resulting increase in weight bearing. In this type of pool, however, only a limited area of the water is sufficiently deep to give the maximum effect of buoyancy and the patient cannot move so freely over the pool as a whole.

For Bad Ragaz techniques (see Chapter 7) the floor must be level so that the physiotherapist is working in a depth of 1·1 m approximately. If the pool is very large and the techniques can be performed from one side to the other the pool floor can be graded. Where Halliwick techniques (see Chapter 11) are to be used it is desirable to have a deeper area up to 1·42 m as well as a shallow area of 0·84 m. The shallow area is advisable if children are to walk in the pool, but the deeper area is useful for some advanced activities, e.g. somersaults.

Use of a bay is an alternative method of varying the depth of a pool, a free-standing rectangular pool being extended to give one, or more, shallow bays, each to accommodate one patient for exercise. The bays are usually 1·83–2·44 m wide and 0·46–0·84 m deep. They may be used as an introduction to pool therapy in cases where the hydrostatic pressure of deeper water could cause respiratory distress, or to give the physiotherapist good control of a very nervous patient.

TANKS

A tank which may be installed where space is limited is usually trefoil or keyhole shaped, 2·89 m long, 2·08 m across at its widest point with a depth of water of 0·76 m. The wings allow for arm movements. The patient can be treated on the stretcher on which he is lifted into the tank, and, as the rim of the tank is waist high, it is easy for the therapist to handle the patient. The water can be changed after each patient, as is necessary in the treatment of burns or septic conditions.

Douche. To provide local treatment for stiff joints and muscular spasm, an underwater jet from a flexible tube can be installed. This operates at a temperature 6°C (10°F) above that of the pool and at a pressure of 7000 kg/m². It is unfortunately less easily fitted to pools controlled by circulatory plant, but could be a useful adjunct to treatment.

HANDRAILS

Whatever the type of pool, it is surrounded by a handrail made of stainless steel, plastic-coated metal or of teak approximately 40 mm in diameter and fixed 50–80 mm from the pool wall, at water level.

An additional rail is desirable 240–300 mm below the water level. There must also be handrails on both sides of the steps leading into and out of the pool.

METHODS OF ENTRY

STEPS

The steps leading to the pool should have 150 mm risers and be 300 mm in depth. The width of the steps should be 600 mm so that both the rails can be easily grasped. If the pool is of the raised type there should be a small platform at the top and a second flight of stairs leading down to floor level.

The front edge of each step should be clearly marked by, for example, different-coloured tiles.

RAMP

Where there is sufficient space and many wheelchair patients are to be treated, a ramp may be installed so that disabled patients can be wheeled directly into the water. A very shallow gradient is essential for safety.

OVER THE SIDE

Children may enter over the side as indicated in the chapter on the Halliwick method. Where there is a raised pool a patient may transfer from a wheelchair to the edge of the pool, swing the legs over, with or without assistance, then enter the pool.

HOISTS

A hoist is required to lift handicapped patients in and out of the pool. This may be electrically, pneumatically or hydraulically powered; the mechanical types are not used so frequently nowadays. The hoist should be designed so that it can be worked by one operator who is positioned to control the patient while the hoist is in use. There are four chains permanently fixed to the hoist at one end, and the free ends are clipped each time to the sling, chair or stretcher. A specially designed sling carrying the patient in a reclined sitting posture may be used as the patient feels secure in this position and the wheelchair used with it takes up less space than a stretcher. The wheelchair in which the patient is taken through the shower to the hoist must be capable of standing up to water.

FOOTBATH

All people entering the pool have to immerse their feet in a solution of chlorinated water (100 ml Voxsan per 5 litres of water) and this is provided by a footbath placed near to the steps (Fig. 2.4); it is best built into the floor with its own taps and drainage.

For patients entering by wheelchair or over the side there must be a small plastic tub in which the patients' feet can be immersed.

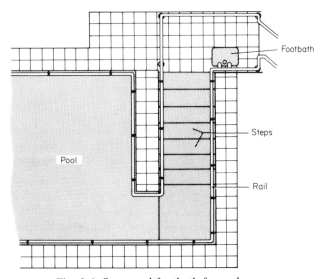

Fig. 2.4. Steps and footbath from above.

POOL AREA

SIDEWALKS

The sidewalks surrounding the pool are at least 1·22 m wide on three sides and 2·44 m or more on the fourth side where the hoist and steps are placed, and there is room for stretchers and chairs. Slip-proof, ridged or studded tiles are used for the flooring, which is very slightly sloped to allow effective drainage of surplus water.

For the safety of both patients and therapists there should be a handrail on the wall 850 mm above the sidewalk. This is useful not only as a grabrail, but also in encouraging patients to keep well away from the pool edge.

If the sidewalk is wide enough (2·44 m) a non-enclosed shower may be installed. This is useful for patients and staff showering just prior to entering the pool.

LIGHTING AND VENTILATION

The pool area should be well lit, preferably by natural light, and designed to give a feeling of spaciousness. Ideally, windows should be double glazed, made of frosted glass and positioned so that sunlight will not dazzle the patient during treatment. The pool area is usually kept at 25°C (78°F), and the changing and rest rooms at 21°C (70°F). Ventilation should prevent too much condensation, and to this end, the ceiling and walls have a special surface. Humidity is kept at 50–60%. It has been found that condensation occurs when heating is turned off in the hydrotherapy department at the weekend.

ALARM AND FIRST AID EQUIPMENT

All pool areas should be fitted with an alarm system which can be triggered by a physiotherapist in the pool, for example with red cords hanging at arm's length above the surface of the water (Fig. 2.2). The system should have a distinctive noise and flashing lights may also be incorporated. All staff must be trained to recognize these emergency signals.

First aid equipment may include sticking-plaster, Micropore or Op-Site and sterile dressings. There should be a Brook's Airway readily available. Other emergency equipment such as an Ambu Bag and resuscitation tray may be available depending upon the site of the pool and the policy agreed by the physiotherapists, doctors and administrators of the hospital.

POOL EQUIPMENT

PARALLEL BARS

Parallel bars are useful for patients performing leg, arm and trunk exercises as well as for walking practice. The height of the bars should be adjustable to within 700–800 mm from the floor and the width approximately 700 mm. They must be absolutely stable, but may be movable. A bench with slatted back, placed with the back

700–750 mm from the wall, may be used to form one bar whilst the handrail forms the second bar.

Stretchers or plinths for use in the pool are best made of tubular steel with a nylon mesh cover and can be hooked on to the rail of the pool. A full-length stretcher can be supported on a platform at the far end. A half-length stretcher supports itself against the pool wall; in each case the angle of the stretcher can be adjusted. The half stretcher is generally more useful, giving freedom for lower-limb exercises and taking up less space.

The patient is secured to the stretcher by adjustable straps made from 80-mm webbing (1·2–1·5 m in length) with 450-mm Velcro fastening at each end.

The stools and benches are made from teak, and are weighted to keep them on the pool floor. Stools of varying heights should be available to keep the shoulders of patients of all heights immersed.

An inflated semicircular ring is used to support the head of the patient in floating.

Floats are made of cork or polystyrene. Blocks (300 × 150 × 150 mm) attached to each end of a canvas sling may be used to support the trunk. Smaller blocks or balls with a length of cord through the centre are used as supports for the limbs, or for added resistance in downward movements. An 80-mm polystyrene block provides a resistance of 0·5 kg when pushed down against buoyancy.

Rubber rings are available in diameters ranging from 300 to 600 mm and they can be used for trunk or limbs.

Bats with diameters of 120, 180 and 240 mm are useful for progressive exercises. Used horizontally they will give a stream-lined effect, and when used vertically and with increasing size there will be a greater resistance to movement. Flippers can be used for the feet.

A weighted raised sandal for a patient with legs of unequal length is useful for practice walking. Crutches or sticks will require weight at the base to overcome buoyancy. Splints made of polystyrene or perspex are useful for applying to a patient to support an unstable limb.

Floating toys may be used when children are being treated.

Equipment not made of rubber should be stored on slatted wooden shelves. Rubber floats are best stored by being suspended on wooden pegs projecting from the wall of the storage room. The canvas of the stretchers will rot if they are left in the pool all the time, so they should be taken out when they are not in use.

UTILITIES

SHOWERS
As all the staff and patients must take a shower before entering the pool the shower should be sited close to the pool. The shower cubicle should be large enough to take a wheelchair or stretcher. The spray head of the shower should be fixed to a tiled wall 1·5 m up and angled so that the water does not necessarily wet the hair. A flexible tube and spray head should also be available for chair patients. The temperature of the water must be thermostatically controlled. Handrails are fixed on all walls. The floor, which is made of a non-slip tile, should have a fall to allow water to drain quickly to flush-type gullies.

CLOTHING AND LINEN
It is more practical to provide a specially designed swimsuit, especially if patients require assistance with changing. Trunks or pants with a side opening, secured by Velcro, and a bra top, also secured by Velcro, are much easier to put on and remove than a regulation-type swimsuit.

The patient will also need to be provided with a towelling dressing gown, cap and pair of slippers. The slippers need to stand up to soaking in disinfectant; a type frequently used is made of rubber and has straps across the forefoot. After treatment a large (1·5 × 2·0 m) turkish towel or twill sheet is required. Blankets and pillows will be necessary for the couch.

The physiotherapist must also be provided with costume, cap, slippers and dressing gown.

Between treating patients, the physiotherapist may be required to leave the pool. In this case, she should wrap herself in a warm twill sheet and put a turkish towelling dressing gown on top. The sheet may be applied safely and securely if it is first placed lengthways across the physiotherapist's back, just below the axillae—clearing the ground. The two top corners are then brought forwards under the arms, crossed in front and then tied behind the neck.

CHANGING, REST, UTILITY AND LINEN ROOMS

Adequate space must be allotted for patients to change and rest. Whilst some patients can manage in a cubicle with a seat and locker, disabled patients need to change in a cubicle furnished with a couch.

Each rest cubicle should be furnished with a 2-m wooden couch, 500 mm high with a 100-mm-thick plastic-covered mattress. As more people will be using the cubicles than are in the pool at one time, sufficient cubicles are essential.

Lavatories and wash basins should be nearby. They should be large enough to take wheelchair patients and be fitted with handgrips.

A separate staff changing room should be provided which is equipped with shower, lavatory, wash basin and clothes lockers.

The utility room is fitted with a sink and draining boards and with slatted shelves along one wall (for drying equipment such as floats). An industrial washing machine and spin dryer will most probably be required for washing the swimsuits. Space is required for containers with sterilizing solution in which caps and slippers may be soaked. A suitable solution is 100 ml Voxsan in 13·5 litres of water. Shoes are soaked for 15 minutes and then washed down, while caps are soaked for 5 minutes before rinsing.

A well-heated linen room fitted with slatted shelves will be required to store the clothing and linen.

Whilst the physiotherapists are concerned with treating the patients, aides should attend to the patients' other needs and assist with their changing of clothes. They will also be responsible for looking after the linen and the washing of costumes, slippers etc.

In training schools students should know these duties, and it is important that they should understand what their responsibilities will be, and what is involved in the running of a hydrotherapy department.

WATER TEMPERATURE AND PURIFICATION

The temperature at which the pool is kept is influenced by the general atmospheric conditions and the ventilation of the department as a whole. Humidity increases as the water temperature rises, and this can prove fatiguing for patients and staff. Pool temperatures vary from 34 to 37°C (94–98°F), according to the specific need. For cases of orthopaedic and spinal injury, the pool is usually between 34 and 36°C (94–96°F), whereas arthritic conditions are treated more satisfactorily at a temperature of 36–37° (96–98°F). Thermometers and hygrometers should be available in the department so that water and air temperatures and the humidity can be tested.

A plant is required for heating, filtering, sterilizing and exchanging the water. This is designed to give a complete water turnover every 4 hours or less.*

From the pool outlet the water passes through a coarse strainer before being pumped into the filter, and circulated through the calorifier, which heats the water to the desired temperature; finally, the sterilizing agent is added. The water is aerated by passing it through a closed chamber into which air is blown—this helps to maintain bacterial purity and gives a sparkle to the water.

A procedure known as a backwash should be carried out daily in order to flush the filter clean. The water supply to the pool is closed off and water is made to pass rapidly backwards through the filter by a special system of valves and taps. Responsibility for this lies with the maintenance engineer.

Each year, the pool should be emptied and cleaned.

The chlorination of the water should give a result of 0·5–1·5 parts per million of free chlorine, too high a concentration acting as an irritant to the skin. Alum and the chlorine used for sterilization and coagulation are acid-forming, and as water purified by continuous filtration should be kept slightly alkaline with a pH value of 7·2–8·0 it is necessary to add an alkali such as soda ash or lime to the water before it reaches the sand filter. Should it become too alkaline, hydrochloric acid is added.

The residual chlorine content and pH value are tested two or three times throughout the day, and, in addition, a bacteriological analysis of the water is made every 2 weeks. Regular chlorine testing is necessary because some evaporates, some adheres to the body surface and the addition of any water dilutes the concentration of chlorine.

The physiotherapist can check the residual chlorine by using a simple apparatus based upon the orthotolodine test. This apparatus

*See 'Purification of Swimming Baths', HMSO.

consists of two test tubes, a holder and a test tablet of diethyl phenylene diamine (DPD) No. 1 (for free chlorine). The physiotherapist fills both tubes with pool water and places them in the holder. On one side of the holder there is a chart which can be turned to produce different colours in front of one test tube and the tablet is put into the other tube which is then shaken thoroughly. The physiotherapist turns the chart until the colour is the same as that produced by the tablet and the reading is recorded.

The physiotherapist should keep a daily log recording the hours for which the plant is working, the number of people using the pool, and the results of the checks on the chlorine content and pH of the water. From this record can be calculated the amount of chlorine and alkali to be added to the water to maintain its purification.

If the pool is without sterilizing plant, the chlorine is added directly at regular intervals during the day. Bromine is used in some pools instead of chlorine for disinfecting—it is less pH dependent than chlorine and there appears to be less eye irritation.

THE HEALTH AND SAFETY AT WORK ACT 1974

As in all physiotherapy departments, the requirements of this Act must be meticulously adhered to in the hydrotherapy department. In accordance with the Act, employers have a responsibility to produce a written policy which in a physiotherapy department is often prepared and implemented by the Head of Department and the Safety Representative. Staff are required to read the general policy and understand its particular implications to them. The Head of Department and Safety Representative should carry out inspections every 3 months to ensure that the policy is adhered to and updated regularly. These inspections should take only 15 minutes in a hydrotherapy department, and accurate records must be kept. They are valuable in ensuring safety of equipment, which benefits both patients and staff.

Safety precautions
Before a patient is considered for pool treatment all contraindications as described in Chapter 4 should be ruled out. Dangers relating to the patients during treatment, for example accidents and infection, and precautions necessary, are recorded in Chapter 5.

The general procedure as stated in Chapter 6 should be strictly followed before, during and after treatment.

Pool equipment

The safety inspections must include checking of all equipment including floats, rings and stretchers. Any punctures should be repaired and if the rubber has perished the equipment must be replaced. The attachments of permanent fixtures should be checked and any wooden apparatus should be made of hard wood, for example teak, and checked for splinters. Hoists and wheelchairs must be regularly oiled and checked for any loose screws. Any equipment not in regular use must be tested before being used to treat patients. The alarm bell, like the fire bell, should be tested weekly. The pool, its surrounds and rest room must have a set cleaning programme with daily, weekly and monthly routines. Dressing gowns, swimming costumes, towels or sheets should be used only once and then washed. Blankets should be changed weekly. The pool around the water line should be scrubbed with a cleaning agent or surgical spirit and the floor of the surrounds swilled down daily.

Disinfectants and cleaning substances

Chemicals which are used for disinfecting or cleaning the pool or its equipment should be handled with care and stored separately in a cool dark place in their original containers. It may be necessary to dilute them before application; therefore spillage must be avoided and, if it occurs, the chemical should be swabbed or washed away with water. Goggles and gloves should be worn for protection when chemicals are being handled. In the event of fire, the fire brigade should be informed of the types of chemicals. If the pool is chlorinated by hand, the disinfectant should be added in small quantities in several different places but never while there are people in the water. Bacteriological tests should be done every 2 weeks, but the chlorine and pH value are tested daily.

Staff

There should always be at least two people within the pool area when patients are being treated in the pool. A routine must be established for removing a patient from the pool quickly and all staff must be instructed in the first-aid procedures for cardiac arrest, sudden submersion or acid burns, with a knowledge of where the relevant equipment is stored.

Two sessions of one and a half hours' duration in the pool with 20- to 30-minute intervals should be considered as reasonable for each therapist to undertake daily, but initially shorter sessions might be necessary.

3

Physiological and Therapeutic Effects of Exercise in Warm Water

The physiological effects of pool therapy combine those brought about by the hot water of the pool with those of exercise, but the extent of such effects varies with the temperature of the water, the length of the treatment and the type and severity of the exercise. The average temperature of the water in the pool is 35·5–36·6°C (96–98°F) and the immersion period for most patients is 20 minutes, although some patients may begin with as little as 5 minutes or may stay in for as long as 45 minutes.

PHYSIOLOGICAL EFFECTS

DURING IMMERSION

During the period of immersion the physiological effects are similar to those brought about by any other form of heat but are less localized. A general rise in body temperature frequently occurs owing to several factors. The temperature of the water is above that of skin temperature, which is normally 33·5°C (92–93°F). The body therefore gains heat through the areas under water, but can lose it only from the blood in the cutaneous vessels and the sweat glands of the exposed areas, such as the face and neck. The body gains heat from the water and from muscular energy conversion during exercise. A rise in body temperature is therefore inevitable, the rise varying from patient to patient.

As the skin becomes heated the superficial blood vessels dilate and the peripheral blood supply is increased. The blood flowing through these vessels is heated and, by conduction, the temperature of the underlying structures (such as muscles) rises, their vessels dilate and their blood supply increases. This results in a redistribution of blood and the splanchnic vessels constrict to supply the increased volume of blood to the periphery. The heart rate increases with the temperature rise and as a result of exercise, the increase being proportional to the temperature of the water and the severity of the exercise.

As the patient enters the pool the cutaneous vessels constrict momentarily, causing a rise in peripheral resistance and a momentary rise in blood pressure. During immersion the arterioles dilate, producing a reduction in peripheral resistance and therefore a fall in blood pressure.

A rise in temperature increases metabolism; therefore metabolism in the skin and muscles is increased and, as the body temperature rises, so does the general metabolic rate. This increases not only the demand for oxygen but also the production of carbon dioxide, causing the respiratory rate to increase in proportion.

The relatively mild heat of the water reduces the sensitivity of sensory nerve endings, and as the muscles are warmed by the blood passing through them their tone will diminish.

In the skin, there is blanching due to the vasoconstriction and this is followed by pinkness and then redness due to the dilatation. There is increased activity of sweat and sebaceous glands as the skin temperature rises. Long contact with water macerates keratin which, by absorption of water, becomes soft, thick and white.

AFTER IMMERSION

When the patient leaves the pool the heat loss mechanism comes into operation and the temperature returns to normal, owing chiefly to the considerable activity of the sweat glands; this results in considerable fluid loss from the body. Immediately after treatment the patient is wrapped in a warm absorbent sheet and blankets that restrict heat loss from the surface capillaries but encourage sweating. After the rest period the patient will continue to lose heat from the sweat glands and from the surface vessels. While the patient is resting, the heart, respiratory and metabolic rates, and distribution of blood, return to normal. As long as the peripheral arterioles remain dilated and the peripheral resistance remains low, the blood pressure too will be low, but this gradually returns to normal when the vessels constrict during the rest period.

EXERCISE

The physiological effects of exercise in water are similar to those of exercise on dry land. The blood supply to the working muscles is increased, heat is evolved with each chemical change occurring during the contraction, and the muscle temperature rises. There is an increased metabolism in the muscles resulting in a greater demand for oxygen and increased production of carbon dioxide. These changes augment the similar changes brought about by the heat of the water, and both contribute towards the final effects.

THERAPEUTIC EFFECTS

The therapeutic effects of exercise in water are (a) relief of pain and muscle spasm; (b) relaxation; (c) maintaining or increasing the range of joint movement; (d) re-education of paralysed muscles; (e) strengthening of muscles and developing their power and endurance; (f) improving functional activities of walking; (g) increasing the circulation and, thus, the condition of the skin; and (h) boosting the patient's morale by recreational activities and giving the patient confidence to achieve maximum functional independence.

The warmth of the water in which the patient is immersed helps to relieve pain, reduce muscle spasm and induce relaxation. As the pain is relieved, the patient is able to move with greater comfort and the range of joint movement increases. As the warmth of the water also dilates the surface vessels and increases the blood supply to the skin, the condition of the skin improves, particularly in patients with poor peripheral circulation. As the warm blood reaches the underlying muscles and their temperature rises, they contract more easily and with improved function. Similar effects are produced by applying other forms of heat such as infra-red radiation, but the advantage of the pool is that the heat is maintained throughout the exercise, and the muscles become fatigued less quickly although general fatigue may be greater.

The buoyancy of the water supports the body and counterbalances much of the effect of gravity. This support helps to induce relaxation and to relieve pain: the feeling of weightlessness allows the patient to move his joints more freely and with less effort than if he performed the same movement on land. Combined with the effects of heat, buoyancy enables a greater range of movement to be achieved. A heavy patient, who is difficult to move on land, can be moved more easily and with less discomfort in the pool. The equal pressure of water on all aspects on the submerged body will support it in the upright position. This support, together with the 'weight relief' of buoyancy, will give confidence to a patient who has difficulty walking and may indeed enable him to walk in the pool before he can walk on dry land.

A finely graded progression of exercise can be obtained by using buoyancy first to assist movement, then as a support, and finally as a resistance. Each variation of the exercise may be modified by the use of floats, by altering the length of the weight-arm of the part being moved, by changing the speed of the movement and by creating turbulence. As a result of this fine grading a suitable exercise can be selected for any strength of muscle, especially those that are very weak. As muscle power increases the exercises can be progressed so that maximum response is obtained from the muscles.

Recreational activities can be provided by swimming. The different strokes use a wide variety of muscles, and many patients who are severely handicapped out of water are surprisingly mobile in the pool. Apart from the mobilizing and strengthening effects, this is of great psychological value.

Following pool treatment, either later that day or the following morning, the patient may experience more stiffness in treated joints but this usually wears off during normal activities. If the joints continue to ache, and this can occur with rheumatoid joints or joints mobilized after surgery, the treatment has been too vigorous and requires modification.

4

Advantages and Indications, Disadvantages and Contraindications

Exercises in water have their place in the rehabilitation of a patient. Care is required in the selection of patients, and there must be a meticulous examination to determine the stage of the condition and the overall objectives of physiotherapy. As a general rule, where a physiotherapist can justifiably predict that a patient would benefit equally from dry land or pool treatment, the modality of choice is dry land. This is because pool treatment is more time-consuming and more expensive.

ADVANTAGES AND INDICATIONS

The warmth of the water helps to relieve pain and reduce muscle spasm; thus the patient is warm throughout the treatment. This is useful because a number of joints are heated at the same time in a generalized condition such as rheumatoid arthritis, and the warming of the joints and muscles is continued throughout the exercise programme. These effects are also useful for conditions such as osteoarthritis of the hips and knees, ankylosing spondylitis, painful backs and recent injuries affecting large muscles, e.g. hamstring or calf muscle tears.

The force of buoyancy can provide complete support for the body, resulting in effects which are not possible on dry land.

Relaxation can be promoted in free floating because there is no localized pressure on bony prominences. This is useful in the conditions mentioned above. The freedom of movement in floating helps to increase the range of movement without the resistance of friction, which is so difficult to overcome on dry land; e.g. where the pelvis is fixed, trunk side-flexion can be mobilized. Buoyancy also provides weight relief, which is of particular value in treating patients with bilateral osteoarthritis of the hips or recently healed lower-limb fractures. The weight relief obtained is dependent on the proportion of the body below water level. If the head and neck only are out of the water, approximately 90% of the body weight is relieved. This permits walking re-education to start much earlier than on dry land.

The force of gravity is counterbalanced by buoyancy, and therefore some exercises, which require muscles to work against gravity on land, become much easier if performed in the pool because buoyancy assists the movement (e.g. transfers from a bench to a stool). This may help neurological patients. When muscles need to be strengthened buoyancy may be used to provide finely graded exercises, as in progressing from buoyancy-assisting to counterbalanced, to resisting, to the addition of floats (see Chapter 6). Thus pool treatment is especially useful where patients have a large number of weak muscles, e.g. with polyneuritis. Pool therapy is also useful for improving or maintaining muscle strength prior to surgery, as in patients waiting for joint replacements.

An exercise programme can be devised incorporating a large number of joints and muscles, including movements in different planes with minimal alteration of starting position. This is very useful for arthritic, neurological or elderly patients who may find it difficult or painful to move on a dry land plinth.

Disabled patients are more easily moved by the physiotherapist in water than on dry land. This is an advantage in treating tetraplegia, paraplegia and overweight patients.

The freedom of movement provides enjoyment and boosts morale because patients can achieve activities which may not be possible on dry land. This is especially applicable to patients with multiple sclerosis and hemiplegia, and to severely disabled children. Recreational activities and competitive games aid rehabilitation, especially in children. Swimming is valuable for paraplegic patients and underwater swimming is especially useful for patients with ankylosing spondylitis.

DISADVANTAGES

Pool therapy has its disadvantages. The installation and upkeep of pools is expensive; staff costs are also high, especially when one considers that pool treatment has most often to be given on an individual basis and there is a limit to the length of time which both the patient and the physiotherapist can remain in the pool. In addition, the patient sufficiently disabled to need pool treatment will often need transport and help in changing. The ambulance services in this country are second to none in providing emergency help, but they cannot be expected to provide a taxi service as good as that offered by private enterprise. The patient is therefore often late in arriving at the pool and already tired.

It is sometimes difficult to achieve a firm fixation, and so isolation of movement. A constant watch has to be kept on the chlorination of the water and the possible spread of infection. Some patients are afraid of the water, while others may become dependent on it because they can achieve functions in it which they cannot achieve on dry land. Final rehabilitation is extremely difficult in the pool and all patients should complete this on dry land.

Nevertheless the benefits of pool therapy far outweigh the disadvantages, and many patients not only gain physically from this form of treatment but also enjoy the exercise and are loath to stop even when their course of treatment is completed.

CONTRAINDICATIONS

As with any modality of physical therapy there are some absolute contraindications to pool therapy and some instances where caution is necessary.

Absolute contraindications are skin infections, tinea pedis being the most common, but also including ringworm. Since the warm water provides a good medium for bacterial growth, all infections should be considered as contraindications, including ear boils, sore throats, influenza and gastrointestinal infections. Water-borne infections such as typhoid, cholera, poliomyelitis and dysentery are also contraindicated, as are infectious diseases especially related to children.

Patients with a vital capacity of less than 1 litre can be treated in the pool but must be thoroughly assessed, and careful selection of treatment programme is required for those with a vital capacity between 1·0 and 1·5 litres. Evidence of peripheral vascular disease or incipient cardiac failure should be considered an absolute contraindication, as should recent deep X-ray therapy and kidney diseases where the patient cannot adjust to fluid loss. Perforated ear drums may well be a contraindication as it is difficult to avoid splashing.

No hard or fast rules can be given about other conditions and the physiotherapist must rely on her assessment of examination findings. Points to bear in mind are:

(a) Incontinence of faeces would be undesirable, and urinary incontinence would be dealt with prior to entry by manual expression, spigotting of catheter or increased pool chlorination.

(b) Epileptics are not suitable unless well controlled.

(c) Patients with a past history of cardiac disease or high or low blood pressure may be treated for short periods with frequent rests between exercises.

(d) Verrucae, open wounds or ulcers may be covered by verruca socks or Op-Site.

(e) There is no underlying physiological reason for menstruation to be considered as a contraindication, but it is impractical in cases of very heavy flow.

(f) The patient who is frightened of water is unlikely to do well in the pool.

5
Dangers and Precautions

ACCIDENTS

An accident is always possible when a patient undergoes physio-therapy in any form, but such mishaps can be avoided if the physiotherapist is aware of the possible causes of accidents and takes sufficient care to ensure that they do not happen. In hydrotherapy there are hazards additional to those encountered elsewhere in the department, and some of them could produce serious accidents. It is important, therefore, that everyone working in hydrotherapy should be fully aware of possible dangers.

UNEXPECTED SUBMERSION

Unexpected submersion in water is an alarming experience for anyone, and should this occur when a patient is receiving hydrotherapy it could destroy completely his confidence in this form of treatment, particularly if he is at all apprehensive of water.

It could occur while the patient is actually in the pool or during entry or exit. While in the pool, the patient could slip and overbalance, although this danger is reduced in modern pools by the use of non-slip tiles. The patient might be knocked over by another patient. This is most likely to happen if the pool is overcrowded or if a patient is allowed to swim across the pool on his back without making sure that there is a clear space in the water. Care should be taken that the pool does not become overcrowded and—although the number of patients that can be treated at one time will vary with the size of the pool—sufficient space should be available to allow patients and staff to move about freely. Swimming should only be allowed when there is sufficient space available.

Buoyancy may thrust the patient's legs to the surface if floats are carelessly applied or removed. Pelvic rings must be put on over the head when the patient is upright and over the feet only if the patient is already in the lying position.

The effect of buoyancy also allows the patient's legs to float to the surface if he sits down too quickly or too far from the seat. Patients must therefore be warned to stand right back against the stool, to bend the knees and hips, and then to sit down slowly. If a back-rest is available the patient can use it to steady himself.

If a stretcher is used it must be fixed securely to prevent it from sinking under the patient's weight, and should be checked before the patient gets on it.

A handrail round the pool provides the patient with a means of support but the physiotherapist should be in the pool nearby, ready to give help and support if necessary.

In a pool of graded depth it is possible for a patient to walk unexpectedly into deeper water, and for a child to walk beyond his depth. This is more likely in a pool that is graded in steps rather than sloped towards the deep end, but in each instance patients should be warned if the pool is graded. In the former type of pool patients are less likely to mistake the depth of water if different coloured tiles are used to mark the edges of each step.

If the patient enters or leaves the pool by hoist, care must be taken to ensure that he does not fall off it—the chair or stretcher must clear the edge of the pool before being lowered, and the patient's legs must also clear the rim of the pool. If the more rigid type of chair is used, the bar across the front should be securely fastened; however, with the sling-type chair, the patient is less likely to fall as the material of the chair 'moulds' itself to some extent around the patient, so providing extra support. The physiotherapist should be in the pool to receive the patient, as this not only gives him greater confidence but also minimizes the danger of falling as the patient leaves the chair for the water.

When the patient enters the pool by the steps he may lose his footing as he moves from the last step into the pool. The refraction of the water makes it difficult to appreciate when the lowest step is reached, so that, as in the graded pool, the last step should be marked clearly in a different colour; better still, tiles of different colours should be used for all the steps. A handrail on each side of the steps will give the patient support as he enters the pool.

FALLS

Although a patient might fall in any part of a hospital building, the likelihood is greater in the hydrotherapy department, as the floor may be wet and slippery. Falls are most liable to occur on the surrounds of the pool, in the rest room and in the shower cubicle. The patient may also fall over accessory apparatus, such as a float if it is left lying on the floor. To prevent accidents, the tiles on the area around the pool and in the shower are usually ridged or studded, and are unlikely to become slippery. Accessory apparatus should not be left about on the floor or surrounds of the pool. In the shower cubicle a rail fixed to the wall, just less than 1 m from the ground, will minimize the danger of falls. There should also be a similar rail on the walls of the pool room. The floor in the rest room should be covered with studded rubberized material which will not be slippery when it becomes wet. Polished linoleum must be avoided at all costs. Patients and staff must wear non-slip footwear.

These precautions are of particular importance when visually handicapped patients are treated.

A physiotherapist treating children should avoid turning her back on them.

BURNS AND SCALDS

These are infrequent accidents, but they may occur if hot-water pipes are exposed or if a thermostat fails to regulate the temperature of the water in a shower. As a precaution, therefore, all exposed water pipes within the patients' or physiotherapists' reach should be lagged, and thermostats should be checked and overhauled regularly.

PROCEDURE IF AN ACCIDENT OCCURS

Should an accident occur the appropriate measures must be taken without delay.

If a patient becomes submerged in the pool immediate action is required to get his head out of the water. He is taken out of the pool, using a stretcher and hoist if necessary. He should rest on a couch and be wrapped in warm sheets as some degree of shock is likely. If he is badly shocked, distressed, or has injured himself in any way, a doctor must be called to examine him. If he is not badly shocked he may be allowed to rest quietly for half an hour or so, given a hot drink and allowed to go home. All patients who have had an accident of any kind will require help and reassurance from the physiotherapist, but patients who have been inadvertently submerged are naturally frightened by their experience and most will require much encouragement from the physiotherapist before receiving further treatment.

It is also possible, although unlikely, for a patient to drown. In any case in which a patient has been submerged for any length of time, artificial respiration will be required immediately, and a second person should call a doctor. As a precaution in case of accident, there should never be less than two physiotherapists in the department when there is a patient in the pool, and all staff working in the department must be proficient in at least one method of artificial respiration, preferably mouth to mouth breathing, and external cardiac massage. To this end it is advisable to have a Brook's Airway and possibly an Ambu Bag in the department.

Should a patient fall, he must be seen by a doctor before leaving the building. First aid may be given by the physiotherapy staff but the doctor is responsible for subsequent treatment, and must therefore be consulted.

A complete record of all accidents must be made, including treatment given and the names and addresses of any witnesses. These records must be kept for 3 years after the accident occurs, as this is the statutory period during which a patient may institute legal proceedings against the staff and hospital.

UNTOWARD EFFECTS

The physiological changes brought about by exercise in water may result in certain untoward effects of which the physiotherapist should be aware so that she may take the necessary precautions.

A momentary rise in blood pressure occurs as the patient enters the pool; he should therefore enter slowly to minimize this effect and the physiotherapist should remain close to him. While the patient is in the pool his blood pressure falls and will fall still further, gradually returning to normal as he rests afterwards. If the patient assumes the upright position too quickly he may feel dizzy or faint. Therefore he should always get up slowly from any recumbent position, either in the pool or the rest room, and the physiotherapist should always be close to the patient as he stands up.

Chilling may occur if the patient loses heat too quickly by being exposed to a cool atmosphere before the cutaneous vessels have had time to constrict. This can be avoided by giving the patient a shower when he leaves the pool, starting with the water at pool temperature and gradually reducing it to skin temperature, and then wrapping him in a hot sheet and blanket. After the patient is dressed he should be advised to remain in room temperature for 20 minutes or so before leaving the building and, if possible, to have a drink during this time to make good the fluid loss from increased sweating.

Redistribution of blood resulting in constriction of the splanchnic vessels makes it unwise for either patient or physiotherapist to go into the pool much less than an hour after a meal.

The patient or physiotherapist may feel generally fatigued on leaving the pool. Although the reasons for this is uncertain, the rise in temperature, possible cerebral anaemia due to the fall in blood pressure, and an accumulation of metabolites, may be contributing factors. Care should be taken to build up gradually to the maximum time the patient requires in the pool. Similarly, the physiotherapist should not remain continuously in the pool for too long—ideally for not longer than an hour at a time.

Control of humidity, temperature and ventilation contribute to the prevention of these untoward effects (see Chapter 1).

INFECTIONS

All infections or contagious diseases can spread from one person to another in a physiotherapy department, as elsewhere, and the precautions customary in hospitals must be taken by the physiotherapist.

All contagious and infectious skin diseases are a contraindication (see Chapter 4) to pool treatment and patients with such conditions must not be given pool therapy until the skin condition has been cured.

To minimize the spread of infection, the pool is chlorinated regularly, either by a chlorifier incorporated into the circulating mechanism or by adding chlorine manually (see Chapter 2). In addition, a regular bacteriological analysis of the water is carried out. All swimsuits must be washed each time they are used, and all shoes and caps sterilized.

The disinfectant used for sterilizing caps and shoes will vary from one hospital to another. One method is to use a chlorine solution such as Voxsan, 10 ml of which is mixed with 13·5 litres of water. Similarly, dressing gowns, sheets and towels can be used once only before washing. Blankets do not come into contact with the patients but should be changed daily; the cotton cellular type is washed very easily.

There are two conditions which are particularly likely to flourish in the hydrotherapy department and special precautions must be taken against tinea pedis and tinea capitis.

TINEA PEDIS

Tinea pedis is a water-borne fungus infection and may spread very rapidly in such places as swimming pools and hydrotherapy departments. There are two types, the vesicular and the intertriginous. The vesicular type grows on the corneal layer of the skin but may produce changes in the underlying epidermis, causing vesicle formation. This type of infection frequently begins under the arch of the foot and spreads to the heel and even the dorsum of the foot. It is characterized by an erythema under which the vesicles can be seen, first as small white spots but later as purulent vesicles. The infection may be unilateral or bilateral. The intertriginous type begins between the toes, usually the fourth and fifth, and may spread to the other toes and adjacent parts of the sole of the foot. The skin appears white and soft and then peels off, leaving a reddened area beneath.

As the condition is highly contagious every care should be taken to prevent its spread. All patients' feet should be examined at every treatment session, and if there are any signs of infection the patient should not be allowed into the pool. Neither patients nor staff should be allowed to walk anywhere in the department without shoes which should be worn once only and then sterilized in a chlorous solution before being used again. Outdoor shoes should not be worn in the pool area. A footbath containing chlorous solution should be kept at the entry into the pool and everyone should immerse their feet before going into the water. One hundred millilitres of Voxsan is put in a bath containing 13·5 litres of water.

TINEA CAPITIS

Tinea capitis (ringworm) is now relatively rare in the United

Kingdom, but infections do occur and can spread rapidly if proper precautions are not taken. Swimming caps used by patients and staff must be sterilized immediately after use in a chlorous or other disinfectant solution. However, most staff, and many patients, prefer to use their own bathing caps, and these need not be sterilized.

6

Principles of Treatment Part I—Theory

GENERAL PROCEDURE

The physiotherapist must examine the patient thoroughly and having decided that hydrotherapy is the modality of choice must ensure that all contraindications peculiar to hydrotherapy (see Chapter 4) are ruled out. When the patient enters the pool for the first time further assessment is required to determine the effects of buoyancy and warmth on, for example, the patient's muscle strength, joint range, balance and functional activities. Thereafter the patient must be reassessed at regular intervals both on land and in the water so that a comparison can be made with the initial examination findings and the treatment adjusted accordingly.

Checking is required prior to pool entry at every treatment session for the development of contraindications, particularly tinea pedis, and ear, nose, throat or skin infections.

As with all physiotherapy treatment it is important to keep an accurate record of examination findings, treatment given, and patients' progress.

Before entering the pool the patient is given a brief explanation of the nature of the treatment, including approximate duration of each session, length of course and overall objectives. Any precautions are explained and if he is apprehensive of the water he may gain confidence by watching other patients in the pool.

Immediately prior to entry he is given a shower at a temperature of between 34·5 and 35·5°C (94–96°F) which accustoms him to the temperature of the pool. He then immerses his feet in a 1% chlorous solution to prevent the spread of tinea pedis.

If the patient is able, he can enter the pool by walking slowly down the steps—holding the handrails on each side. If he is at all apprehensive, the physiotherapist should walk backwards ahead of him. If he cannot manage the steps, a hoist can be used, the physiotherapist waiting in the pool to receive him.

The length of treatment varies from 5 to 45 minutes, depending on the age and condition of the patient and the temperature of the water. Elderly patients find the temperature of the water enervating; and in combination with the physical activity, this tends to tire them, so a shorter treatment is given. Such patients usually begin with 5–10 minutes' treatment, increasing in length on subsequent occasions to not more than 20 or 25 minutes. Younger patients normally find that they can tolerate longer periods, up to 30–45 minutes. Patients suffering from conditions such as paraplegia, or an injury, will be able to stay in the pool for longer than patients suffering from systemic diseases, such as rheumatoid arthritis. The length of treatment also depends on the temperature of the pool, which can vary, as desired, from 33 to 37·6°C (92–99°F); and the lower the temperature and the younger the patient, the longer the period of immersion he can tolerate. A young paraplegic patient, for example, can withstand 45 minutes at 33°C (92°F), while an older patient with rheumatoid arthritis may tolerate only 20 minutes at 36°C (98°F).

After treatment the patient is again given a shower at 34·5–35·5°C, partly to cool him down and partly to wash away the chlorinated water. In the shower, the patient's swimsuit is removed, and a dressing gown is put on back to front. The patient then goes through to the rest room accompanied by the physiotherapist. A hot sheet is placed lengthwise on the rest couch, the patient lies down, the dressing gown is removed and the sheet is wrapped around him. Part of the sheet goes between the patient's legs and the remainder of the sheet is so arranged as to prevent skin surfaces from touching. The coverings are completed by two blankets, one of which is on the couch before the patient and sheet are positioned so that the sides can be brought up and over the patient. The second blanket is then placed on top and tucked in loosely round the feet so that hyperextension is prevented. The patient is left to rest for 20–30 minutes and should be supported with pillows where appropriate, suitable for his condition. For example, a patient with a hiatus hernia requires extra pillows under the head and thorax, while a patient with ankylosing spondylitis should lie as flat as possible.

The pack allows the patient to cool slowly, reducing the risk of chilling. During the time the physiological changes resulting from immersion return almost to normal, and the patient can relax after treatment in a good, functional position. The patient dries in the pack and no further drying should be necessary. After getting up and dressing slowly he should sit for a short time in the waiting-room, which is heated to about 21°C (70°F). A warm drink is advisable during this time to replace some of the fluid lost during treatment. A young, fit patient who has, for example, sustained an injury may not need to rest after treatment.

A record of the date of attendance is kept for each patient, other points to note being the temperature of the water, the exercises given, the time for which the patient was in the pool and progressions that were made. If any untoward effect is produced this, also, must be recorded.

It may be advisable to take a patient's blood pressure before, during, and immediately after treatment and at the end of the rest period.

STARTING POSITIONS

A variety of different starting positions is commonly used in the pool and can be adapted to the needs of each patient. A stable starting position is sometimes difficult to achieve in water but some degree of fixation may be achieved by mechanical or manual means.

Starting positions in the pool are derived from three fundamental positions, namely lying, sitting and standing. The term 'support' is used where apparatus or manual support is used.

LYING POSITIONS

Lying (ly;). Floating in the supine position.

Prone lying (pr. ly;). Floating face downwards.

Support lying (sup. ly;). The patient is fully supported on a plinth or stretcher fixed to the rail of the pool at one end and to a support in the pool at the other (Fig. 6.1). Straps can be used to prevent the patient from floating off the plinth, and the head is supported on a small pillow or head-rest. In this position the patient is both reasonably stable and fully supported, and the physiothera-

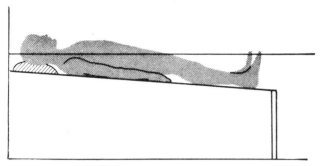

Fig. 6.1. Support lying.

pist has both hands free to assist or resist the movement. There may, however, be some restriction of the patient's knee, hip and trunk movements.

Support side lying (sup. s. ly;). The patient lies on his side on a full stretcher or plinth.

Support prone lying (sup. pr. ly;). This position is adopted on a fixed plinth or on floats, the chin being supported to keep the face clear of the water (Fig. 6.2).

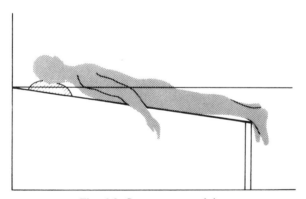

Fig. 6.2. Support prone lying.

Float support lying (fl. sup. ly;). Floats can be used instead to support the patient at the neck, hips, ankles and forearms. This is a comfortable position, especially for patients with spinal deformity, and has the advantage that the physiotherapist can move the patient

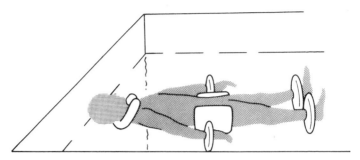

Fig. 6.3. Float support lying.

freely about the pool (Fig. 6.3). Nevertheless, the position is less stable than the plinth method, and fixation of the patient may be more difficult.

Float support side lying (fl. sup. s. ly;). The patient lies on his side supported by floats.

Float support prone lying (fl. sup. pr. ly;). In this position the patient is supported by floats, the chin being supported by a neck float.

Inclined support lying (incl. sup. ly;). In this position the patient lies on a plinth or stretcher which has one end fixed to the rail of the pool, and the other lowered in the water to the required depth (Fig. 6.4).

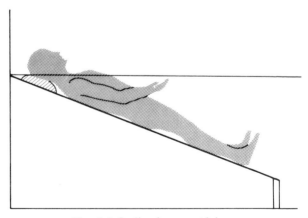

Fig. 6.4. Inclined support lying.

Half support lying ($\frac{1}{2}$ sup. ly;). This position is taken on a half plinth with one end fixed to the rail of the pool, and the other resting against the wall under the rail. The patient's head is supported as before, and floats may be used to support one or both legs. This is comfortable for the patient, and gives him good support and firm fixation; knee and hip movements are unrestricted (Fig. 6.5).

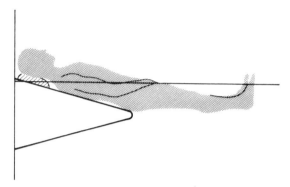

Fig. 6.5. Half support lying.

Half support side lying ($\frac{1}{2}$ sup. s. ly;). The patient lies on his side on a half plinth. He may be fixed by a strap round the pelvis or he may hold the side of the plinth.

Half support prone lying ($\frac{1}{2}$ sup. pr. ly;). In this position the patient lies on a half stretcher, on floats or lies across a full stretcher. Floats are not usually necessary for the legs.

Head support lying (h. sup. ly;). The patient's head is supported on the physiotherapist's shoulder and the pelvis can be supported by a float. This position allows for free movement of all four limbs and thoracic and lumbar spines.

Heave grasp support lying (hve. gr. sup. ly;). The patient grasps the rail above his head with his elbows flexed to 90° and his shoulders abducted to 90°. The pelvis is supported on a float and the head rests on a pillow (Fig. 6.6).

Toe support lying (toe sup. ly,). The patient's toes are fixed under the rail with the feet in dorsi-flexion. The pelvis and neck are supported by floats (Fig. 6.7).

Stretch grasp support prone lying (str. gr. sup. pr. ly;). The patient grasps the rail with the arms stretched above his head. The pelvis is supported by a float (Fig. 6.8).

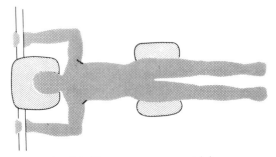

Fig. 6.6. Heave grasp support lying.

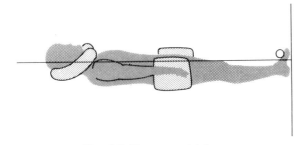

Fig. 6.7. Toe support lying.

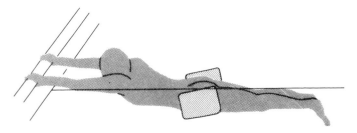

Fig. 6.8. Stretch grasp support prone lying.

SITTING POSITIONS

Sitting (sitt;). In this position the patient sits on a weighted stool or bench with a back-rest (Fig. 6.9). If the bench is slatted the patient can be fixed more easily with straps.

The position is useful for all upper limb movements but care must be taken when the patient has limited or painful shoulder movements to ensure that buoyancy does not thrust the limb into

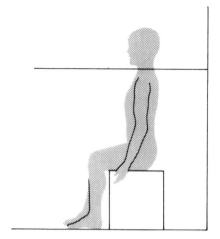

Fig. 6.9. Sitting.

the painful range. It is also useful for trunk rotation, pelvic tilt, knee and ankle exercises, trunk stability and balance.

STANDING POSITIONS

Standing (st;). The patient may stand at the rail, between parallel bars or anywhere in the pool.

Grasp inclined prone standing (gr. incl. pr. st;). The patient faces the rail and grasps it with both hands. He leans forward so that the body is in a straight line and the toes are a suitable distance from the wall (Fig. 6.10).

Half grasp inclined towards side standing ($\frac{1}{2}$ gr. incl. tow. s. st;). The patient stands sideways to the rail and leans towards it, grasping it with the near hand. This is useful for small-range shoulder and hip abduction (Fig. 6.11).

Half grasp inclined away side standing ($\frac{1}{2}$ gr. incl. aw. s. st;). The patient stands sideways to the rail grasping it with the near hand and leans away from it (Fig. 6.12).

Inclined standing (incl. st;). The patient stands with his back to the rail leaning backwards towards it. The head may require a support (Fig. 6.13).

Inclined prone half support standing (incl. pr. $\frac{1}{2}$ sup. st;). The patient leans forward from the hips so that the trunk and the hips are supported on a half stretcher.

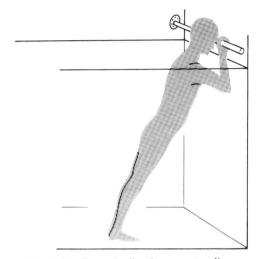

Fig. 6.10. Grasp inclined prone standing.

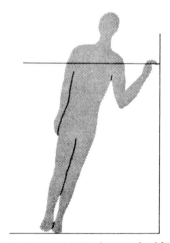

Fig. 6.11. Half grasp inclined towards side standing.

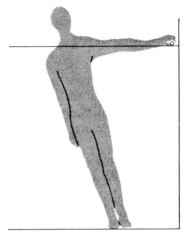

Fig. 6.12. Half grasp inclined away side standing.

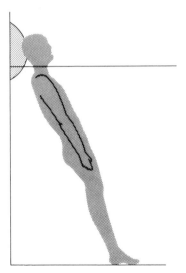

Fig. 6.13. Inclined standing.

OTHER DERIVED POSITIONS

As on land, derived positions from those already described may be used, by positioning the arms or legs; e.g. stretch grasp support lying, or halfyard grasp stride standing ($\frac{1}{2}$ yd. gr. std. st;). The terminology for describing exercises is as on land; e.g. $\frac{1}{2}$ sup. ly;—1L push d. and relax; and $\frac{1}{2}$ yd. gr. s. st;—1Hip and K bend u. and stretch b.

Mechanical fixation. Canvas webbing straps are used to secure a patient to a plinth or stretcher. They have Velcro fastenings.

Manual fixation. This may be by the physiotherapist who fixes the part, e.g. the pelvis to the plinth, or by the patient who may hold the sides of the plinth or pool rail.

PROGRESSION OF EXERCISE

A. STRENGTHENING

A very fine progression of exercise is possible in the pool, making use of the different effects of buoyancy, alteration in the length of the weight-arm of the moving part, and the use of floats. As on land, the rate of progression will depend on the patient's capabilities.

1. *Buoyancy assisting*

A movement is most easily performed when assisted by buoyancy and the part, such as a limb, moves from a position at right angles to the surface of the water to the horizontal position. The effect of buoyancy increases as the part approaches the horizontal, provided it is still immersed, decreasing again if the range of movement is taken beyond it. It is necessary to ensure that the patient himself performs or tries to perform the movement, otherwise the exercise becomes passive.

The progression with buoyancy assisting is made from a long weight-arm to a short weight-arm. The range and difficulty of the movement can be increased by beginning it further from the horizontal position.

2. *Buoyancy as a support*

When buoyancy is used in this way it neither assists nor resists movement of the part. Progression is made from a short weight-arm to a long weight-arm.

3. *Buoyancy resisting*

When buoyancy is used to resist movement, the part is moved against the upthrust of the water from the horizontal position to one at right angles to the surface. If movement is continued beyond this point buoyancy will begin to assist the movement. The effect is greatest as the part moves from the horizontal, and the exercise may be progressed by beginning the movement near to the vertical position and then increasing the range to begin nearer to the horizontal.

The progression with buoyancy resisting is: (*a*) with a short weight-arm; (*b*) with a long weight-arm; (*c*) with a long weight-arm and float, moving the float from the proximal to the distal end of the part; and (*d*) by increasing the size or number of floats.

In each position further progression is brought about by having the part (i) streamlined and moving slowly; (ii) streamlined and moving quickly to increase turbulence; (iii) unstreamlined and moving slowly; (iv) unstreamlined and moving quickly.

As on land, an exercise in water can be progressed by increasing the number of times it is performed or increasing the range of movement; also the physiotherapist may give manual resistance—or assistance—as required.

Strengthening the extensor muscles of the hip

1. The patient is in the prone position on a half plinth or on floats—buoyancy assisting (Figs 6.14 and 6.15).
2. The patient is lying on his side on a half plinth or on floats—buoyancy as a support (Figs 6.16 and 6.17).
3. The patient lies supine on a half plinth or on floats—buoyancy resisting (Figs 6.18–6.21).

A careful record should be kept of the starting position and progression for each muscle. This progression may be adapted to almost any muscle group, depending on the requirements of treatment; and this is implied when reference is made to graded progression in subsequent chapters.

B. MOBILIZING

Exercises for mobilizing joints in the pool should be performed slowly in order to allow full-range movement and minimize resistance due to turbulence. As far as possible the starting position

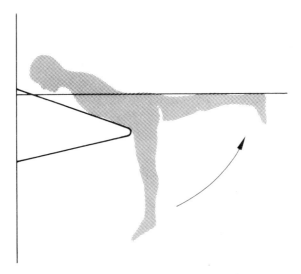

Fig. 6.14. Buoyancy assisting—long weight-arm.

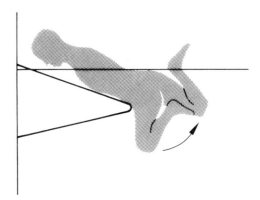

Fig. 6.15. Buoyancy assisting—short weight-arm.

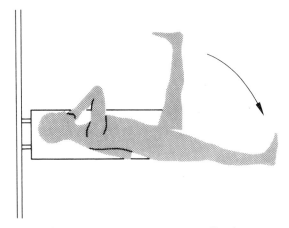

Fig. 6.16. Buoyancy as a support—streamlined movement.

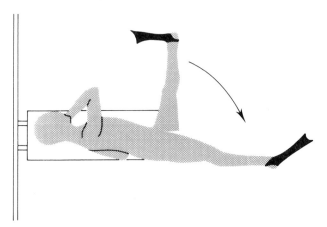

Fig. 6.17. Buoyancy as a support—unstreamlined movement.

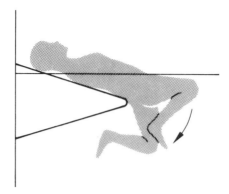

Fig. 6.18. Buoyancy resisting—short weight-arm.

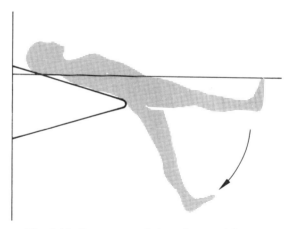

Fig. 6.19. Buoyancy resisting—long weight-arm.

should be such that buoyancy is counterbalanced or assisting throughout the movement. The longer the leverage of the moving part, the more mobilizing the exercise and the patient is encouraged to think of a slow sweeping movement through the water. The range

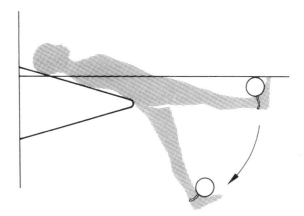

Fig. 6.20. Buoyancy resisting—long weight-arm and small float.

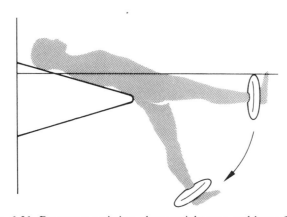

Fig. 6.21. Buoyancy resisting—long weight-arm and large float.

of movement can be increased by either altering the depth of the water in which the exercise is performed or the starting position of the exercise.

In abduction of the shoulder joint the patient can carry out the exercise by sitting on progressively lower seats (Fig. 6.22). The starting position can be changed from 'half grasp inclined towards side standing' to 'half grasp standing' to 'half grasp inclined away side standing'. These positions gradually increase the range of left shoulder abduction (Fig. 6.23).

Fixation is important to localize movement to the affected joints. For example, to increase side-flexion of the trunk the physiotherapist stands between the patient's legs and grasps the pelvis with the patient in float lying.

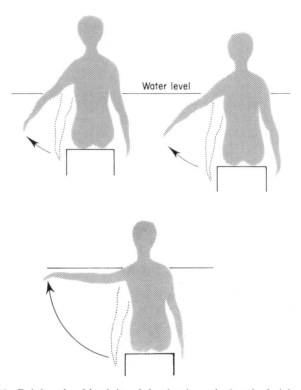

Fig. 6.22. Gaining shoulder joint abduction by reducing the height of the seat.

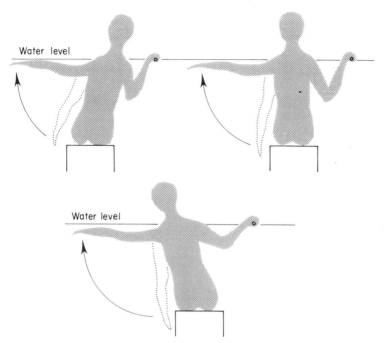

Fig. 6.23. Gaining shoulder abduction by altering the starting position.

C. BALANCING

When a patient is upright in the water both hydrostatic pressure and buoyancy assist in maintaining the trunk in an upright position. Hydrostatic pressure is equal in all directions (see Chapter 1). Slight displacement of the body results in buoyancy, tending to return the body to the vertical position (see Fig. 1.11). Progression of balancing practice is obtained by the physiotherapist creating turbulence around the patient or by the patient creating his own turbulence, at first with hands only and then with bats. If turbulence is created to the right of the patient he will tend to fall to the right side and the muscles on the left side have to work harder to maintain the upright position.

7

Principles of Treatment Part II—Specialized Techniques

'HOLD–RELAX' TECHNIQUE

The 'hold–relax' technique is used to increase the range of movement of a joint, mainly where the limiting factor is muscle spasm. It is applied in the same manner as on dry land but buoyancy may be used to assist in regaining the movement which is limited, and therefore the starting position is chosen accordingly.

For example, to gain flexion of the left knee, the patient is placed in inclined prone lying on a half stretcher and the physiotherapist stands in stride, on the right side of the patient, with her right foot against the patient's right heel, for stability (Fig. 7.1).

The physiotherapist's right hand steadies the left side of the pelvis and her left hand is placed on the anterior aspect of the lower leg. The knee is bent as far as possible in the pain-free range, either actively or passively. At the command 'hold' the physiotherapist applies resistance with the left hand and the knee extensor muscles contract strongly isometrically. At the command 'relax', she releases the resistance and steadies the lower leg as the extensor muscles relax and buoyancy assists further flexion of the knee. The patient may reinforce this by bending the knee actively, and at the same time proprioceptive stimulation may be added by applying resistance to the posterior aspect of the lower leg.

Although it is preferable to have buoyancy assisting the movement into the limited range, this technique may be given with buoyancy neutralized. As on dry land, the movement into the

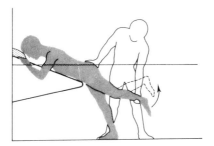

Fig. 7.1. To gain flexion of knee.

limited range may be gained passively, by a free active movement or a resisted movement.

TECHNIQUE OF STABILIZATIONS

This technique can be used in the pool as on land, to obtain a co-contraction of all muscle groups around a joint. In the pool use is made of the freedom of movement. The joint is put in a pain-free position and the physiotherapist's hands are placed just distal to the joint. She then begins by moving the patient in one direction while commanding him to 'hold' the position, and this causes contraction of one group of muscles. Once this muscle group can be felt contracting the physiotherapist moves the patient in a different direction and another group of muscles contract. The direction is altered continually and the movement gradually reduced, thereby reversing the direction more quickly, until the patient is holding his body steady by the co-contraction of all the muscles round the joint.

In Fig. 8.1 (p. 107) this technique can be seen being applied to the knee joint. The patient is in float lying and the physiotherapist grasps the patient's foot and lower leg. When the patient is pushed away the quadriceps contract, and when the patient is pulled back towards the physiotherapist the hamstring muscles contract. At first the patient can be seen to move away and towards the therapist, but this movement is gradually reduced until the patient is holding the knee in a set position by the co-contraction of the quadriceps and hamstring muscles. The technique is useful for maintaining or increasing muscle strength, increasing circulation to painful joints, improving balance and co-ordination.

Key to diagrams in this chapter

▲   Physiotherapist's right hand   ⟶ Patient moves
△   Physiotherapist's left hand   --⟶ Physiotherapist moves
                        ⤳ Turbulence

REPEATED CONTRACTIONS

Repeated contractions are necessary for the learning process and the development of strength and endurance. Repeated activity of the weaker components of a muscle pattern is obtained through a technique of emphasis; a movement is repeated such that the muscle group is worked to maximum capacity. The technique utilizes both isotonic and isometric muscle work. In the pool the patient can move and 'hold' the movement against turbulence alone or turbulence and buoyancy.

An example using turbulence alone—right shoulder abduction
The patient lies supine supported by a neck float and the physiotherapist stands either between the patient's legs or on the right side of the patient, fixing the pelvis in order to move the body to the right. The patient is commanded to move his right arm out then 'hold' the position while he is moved by the therapist in a circle to the right. This is repeated through as full a range as possible (Fig. 7.2). To increase turbulence the patient holds a bat, or is moved faster through the pool

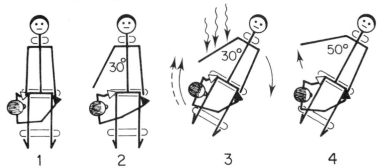

Fig. 7.2. Repeated contractions for right shoulder abductors. 1) Starting position. 2) Push A out sideways. 3) Patient is instructed to hold A—therapist moves patient round to right or clockwise. 4) Patient instructed to move A further out. Stage 5 (not illustrated) Patient holds A steady and therapist moves clockwise again.

An example using turbulence and buoyancy—bilateral leg extensiu..,
abduction and medial rotation

The patient lies supine with the trunk supported on a half stretcher
and floats round the ankles while the physiotherapist places her
hands on the lateral borders of the feet, particularly over the outer
side of the heels. The patient is commanded to turn the legs in, push
down and out and → 'hold' → push down and out → 'hold' again →
'hold' and slowly return to the starting position. The technique can
be repeated with a greater number of floats at the ankles. A quick
manual stretch may be applied immediately prior to the command
'push' to facilitate muscle contraction.

BREATHING EXERCISES

These exercises are used to increase costal expansion, laterally and
posteriorly, and to improve the range of side-flexion and rotation of
the trunk. Vital capacity is therefore increased. In the pool, use is
made of the increased freedom of movement due to relief of pain
and muscle spasm, and support of the body weight by buoyancy.
The starting position is ½ sup. ly. The patient's legs and pelvis are
moved passively to one side to the position where he feels stretched
and the patient is asked to 'breathe deeply into the stretched side in
his own time'.

The therapist has to observe the patient's breathing pattern
carefully and she should not disturb his rhythm. Just before the
inspiration begins, she applies a light stretch with one hand to the
patient's lower limbs, while with the other hand she encourages
more rib movement by applying gentle pressure on the lateral or
posterior aspect of the rib cage.

The stretch on legs is maintained during the length of inspiration,
and only slightly reduced during a calm expiration. The patient is
asked to take several normal breaths, and the procedure is repeated
another two or three times, trying to increase the range of
movement a little bit more each time. Between each set of
exercises, active movements are performed, for example, trunk
side-flexion to avoid overventilation, and to maintain the improved
mobility.

These exercises are very helpful to increase trunk mobility and
vital capacity in patients suffering from ankylosing spondylitis; they
will help reduce spasticity in paraplegia, tetraplegia and hemi-

plegia, as well as maintain mobility and lung function; and they will improve lung excursion and vital capacity in patients with peripheral neuropathies.

Left lateral costal expansion with trunk side-flexion to the right
The starting position is ½ sup. ly; with the patient's legs moved to his right. The therapist's left hand is on the lateral aspect of the patient's left thigh or lower left ankle, and her right hand is on the left side of the patient's thorax (Fig. 7.3). An alternative hand position is illustrated in Fig. 8.4 (p. 114). The patient is asked to breathe in deeply into his stretched left side in his own time. Just before the inspiration begins, a light stretch is applied to the patient's legs, and pressure to the thorax, and both are maintained during the inspiratory phase. The patient relaxes during expiration and then breathes normally. This is repeated two or three times on the same side, and the patient is allowed to perform some active exercises before repeating the breathing exercises on the opposite side.

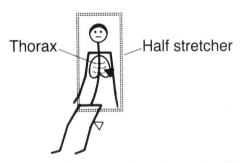

Thorax   Half stretcher

Fig. 7.3. Position to increase left lateral costal expansion. Therapist takes legs to the right and applies manual resistance to the left side of thorax and lateral aspect of left thigh.

Left posterior costal expansion with trunk rotation to the right
The starting position is ½ sup. ly; and both hips and knees are flexed and rolled to the right. The therapist's left hand is on the patient's left knee, and her right hand on the left posterior aspect of the patient's thorax. The exercise continues as above. The stretch can be increased if the lever arm is altered. This is achieved by straightening both knees to the right. Stretch can also be applied on the patient's left hip.

In this and the previous exercise, stretch can also be increased by moving the patient's left arm into the heave grasp position.

BAD RAGAZ TECHNIQUES

A technique of exercise therapy in water has been adapted and developed at Bad Ragaz, Switzerland. This method, differing from that already described, utilizes the properties of water whilst at the same time allowing for normal anatomical and physiological function of joints and muscles.

It also utilizes the patterns of movement which can be used on land but differs from proprioceptive neuromuscular facilitation (PNF) techniques in that resistance is not applied by the physiotherapist. Instead resistance is provided as the body moves through the water; the quicker the movement, the greater the resistance.

Buoyancy is used only for flotation and not as a means of altering resistance to exercise. Resistive or assistive work is given, statically or kinetically, to muscle groups in mass movement patterns allowing movement to occur around all axes of the joints concerned. All components of the muscle groups can therefore be worked, i.e. flexion, extension, abduction, adduction and medial and lateral rotation.

When a body moves or is moved through water, differences in pressure occur around that body (bow-wave formation). There is an increase in pressure at the front and a decrease at the rear of the body, causing water to flow into, and eddies to occur in, the area behind the body, producing turbulence; this has a drag effect. By varying the bow wave, resistance to the movement of the body can be varied, as can the movement in relation to turbulence. In order to have control of the patient and to be able to grade the strength of a movement and the resistance given, the physiotherapist must be in the water with the patient. The physiotherapist is the fixed point about which the patient moves and therefore her stability of stance in the water is of utmost importance. It is difficult to use this technique if the water comes as high as the physiotherapist's axillae. Ideally the water level should reach the therapist's lower thoracic spine, otherwise stability is reduced.

The patient lies in supine, side lying or prone lying positions supported by floats. Usually a horseshoe-shape neck collar and a large body ring or float around the pelvis are required and smaller floats are attached to legs and arms as necessary. The density of all the floats is varied according to the size and weight of the patient and the pattern to be performed. The floats provide support for, and aid correct positioning of, the patient.

Depending on the physiotherapist's manual hold on the patient, different areas can be worked, utilizing mass patterns of movement of limb or trunk. Strong resistance can be given to the stronger components of the movement so that overflow or irradiation occurs to the weaker muscle groups; successive induction, slow reversals and stabilization techniques can all be used. The more proximal or the nearer to the centre of buoyancy the hold of the physiotherapist, the greater will be her control over the movement. With proximal holds the patient feels more secure and it is also possible to control more finely the movement occurring at the potentially painful joint. Distal holds at the end of a limb or trunk allow for greater movement excursion of all joints of the part and for stronger muscle action.

The patterns of movement can be divided into lower limb, upper limb and trunk patterns, but they can also be classified as *isotonic* and *isometric*. In the isotonic movements the patient moves towards or away from the physiotherapist who acts as a fixed point. In the isometric movements the patient holds his limbs in a set pattern while being pushed through the water.

ISOTONIC PATTERNS

LOWER LIMB

Extension–abduction–medial rotation of the hip with knee extension and plantar flexion and eversion of the foot
The patient lies supine supported by neck and pelvic floats and a small float on the resting leg. The physiotherapist stands at the patient's feet, slightly to the side of the extremity to be worked. The hip is flexed, adducted and laterally rotated, the knee is flexed and the foot is dorsi-flexed and inverted. The therapist places one hand on the plantar aspect of the foot and the other hand beneath the thigh or knee. On the command 'point your toes, turn your knee in and push' the patient extends, abducts and medially rotates at the hip, extends at the knee and plantar flexes and everts the foot and

toes. The physiotherapist guides and resists the movement so that all the muscles of the pattern work in sequence from distal to proximal producing a smooth coordinated movement. The therapist provides fixation and leans into the movement as the patient moves away. At the end of the movement, the patient relaxes, the therapist moves towards the patient and the limb is flexed in preparation for the next extensor movement (Fig. 7.4).

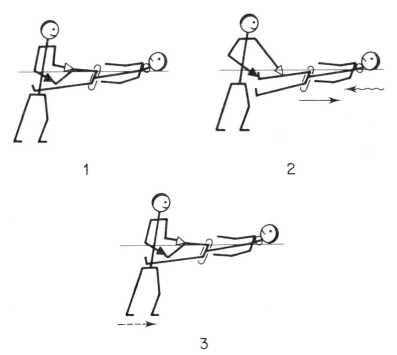

Fig. 7.4. Extension–abduction–medial rotation pattern of the hip. 1) Starting position. Note therapist leans towards patient. 2) Patient extends and moves away from the therapist. 3) Patient relaxes and therapist steps forwards to starting position, bending patient's leg passively.

Flexion–adduction–lateral rotation of the hip with knee flexion, dorsi-flexion and inversion
This is the reverse of the previous pattern. The manual hold of the physiotherapist is now changed and one hand is placed on the dorsal and medial aspect of the foot, the other on the antero-medial aspect of the knee. On the command 'pull your foot up and bend your leg'

the patient moves towards the physiotherapist, who now leans away from the patient to allow full range and adequate movement through the water, thus obtaining the effects of the bow wave. At the end of the movement the patient relaxes, the therapist takes a step backwards and the patient's leg is extended in preparation for the next flexor movement (Fig. 7.5).

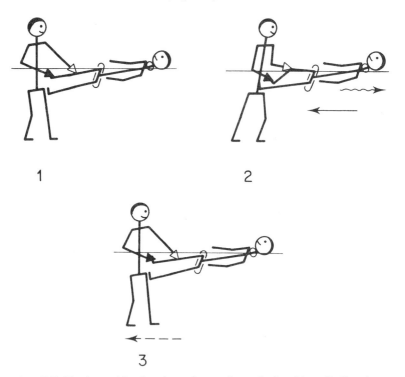

Fig. 7.5. Flexion–adduction–lateral rotation of the hip. 1) Starting position. Note therapist leans away from patient. 2) Patient bends hip and knee and moves through water towards therapist. 3) Patient relaxes, therapist steps back to starting position.

Single-leg abduction pattern
The patient lies supine, supported on floats as previously with a small float around the ankle of the, for example, right leg which is to work isotonically. The physiotherapist stands on the left side of the patient with one hand on the outer aspect of his left foot, the other on the outer aspect of the left thigh resisting isometric work of the

left hip abductors, extensors and medial rotators. The patient is then instructed to push the right leg into abduction with some medial rotation and extension at the hip. As the physiotherapist again leans forward into the movement, an arc should be described in the water by the movement of the patient's right leg. At the end of the movement the patient relaxes, the therapist takes a step forward and moves the left (static) leg towards the right leg in preparation for the movements to be repeated (Fig. 7.6). Care must be taken to ensure that the patient does not side flex the trunk instead of abducting the leg. Also, lateral rotation at the hip must be avoided, otherwise the hip flexors will work and not the hip abductors.

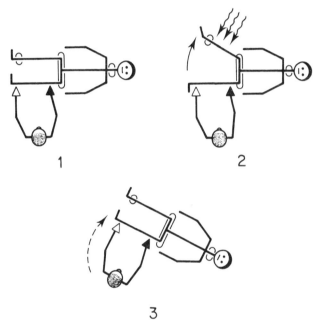

Fig. 7.6. Single-leg abduction. 1) Starting position. 2) Patient abducts right leg. 3) Patient relaxes, therapist moves left leg into starting position. Note that the patient's body has moved round.

Single-leg adduction pattern
This is the reverse of the previous pattern and the patient is in the same float lying position. The therapist changes the manual hold so that the left hand is on the inner aspect of the left foot and the right hand is on the inner aspect of the left thigh.

The patient begins with the right hip in extension, abduction and medial rotation and is instructed to bring the heels together. As the patient brings the legs together the therapist leans away from the movement and moves the point of fixation (i.e. the left leg) further away; thus the patient describes an arc of movement in the water. When both legs are together, at the end of the movement, the patient relaxes, the therapist takes a step back and moves the left (static) leg away from the right leg into abduction and medial rotation in preparation for the movements to be repeated (Fig. 7.7).

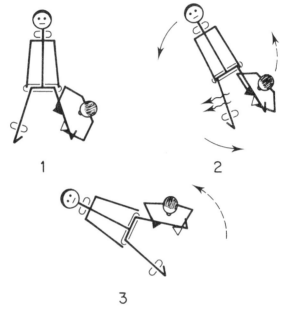

Fig. 7.7. The single-leg adduction pattern. 1) Starting position. Patient has right leg in extension, abduction and medial rotation. Left leg is in abduction. 2) Patient instructed to bring heels together, therapist walks backwards grasping left leg. 3) When legs have come together, patient relaxes, therapist walks backwards grasping left leg and so abducting both legs.

These patterns can be adapted so that both arms and legs are moving. The physiotherapist places one hand on the patient's foot and the other hand on the patient's hand or wrist, resisting isometrically both the arm and the leg while the other arm and leg move into either the extension, abduction and medial rotation pattern or the flexion, adduction and lateral rotation pattern.

Bilateral abduction and adduction patterns
It is often found easier to use these bilateral patterns if the patient's balance in water is poor or if he has a painful hip joint, lacking full range of movement. The patient lies supine with neck float and body float. The physiotherapist stands at his feet and places her hands on the lateral borders of the feet, particularly over the outer side of the heels. The patient abducts both legs, either into extension and medial rotation or into flexion and medial rotation, and the body moves through the water towards the therapist who resists and guides the movement (see Fig. 8.8, p. 122).

During abduction, the therapist stands steady and the patient moves towards her, the patient then relaxes, the therapist steps backwards and passively adducts the patient's legs (Fig. 7.8).

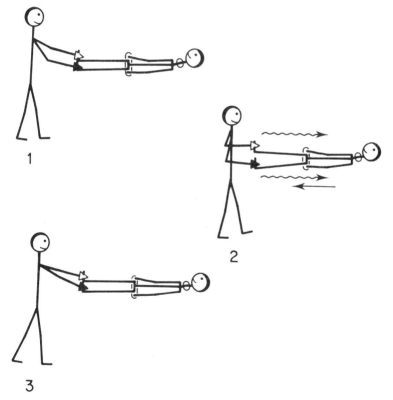

Fig. 7.8. Bilateral abduction. 1) Starting position. 2) Patient abducts. 3) Patient relaxes, therapist steps back.

The pattern is reversed for adduction (Fig. 7.9) and the physiotherapist now places her hands medially over the heels. Adduction occurs with extension with lateral rotation or flexion with lateral rotation.

During adduction, the patient moves away from the therapist, who therefore has to step forward while passively abducting the patient's legs.

It is important that these patterns are performed along the length of the pool and that on adduction, the patient's head is clear of the pool wall.

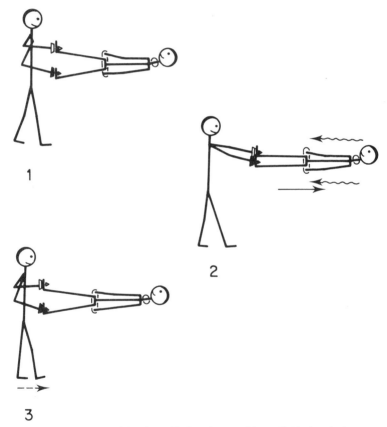

Fig. 7.9. Bilateral adduction. 1) Starting position. 2) Patient's legs are adducted. 3) Patient relaxes, therapist steps forward and abducts patient's legs.

TRUNK
Trunk side-flexion pattern with lower trunk moving
The patient lies supine with neck and pelvic floats and a small float round both ankles. The patient clasps his hands behind his neck, the physiotherapist stands behind his head and places her hands on his elbows.

The patient side-flexes the trunk from side to side while the physiotherapist places one hand under the elbow on the side to which the patient is bending and places her other hand on top of the opposite elbow to give counter-resistance to the movement (Fig. 7.10). Thus the position of the hands is being continually reversed.

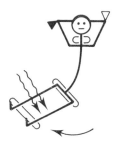

Fig. 7.10. Position of hands during trunk side-flexion to the patient's right.

During the movement, both the physiotherapist and the patient are moving backwards through the water. The patient's arms should be kept on the surface of the water and the physiotherapist must keep her elbows well into her side to avoid side-sway of the patient's trunk.

Pelvic rotation can be added to the movement to emphasize trunk flexion or extension. For trunk extension and movement to the right, the patient turns his pelvis so that the right hip is uppermost and then pulls his legs to the right, the physiotherapist giving counter-resistance to the movement by her pressure at the elbows (Fig. 7.11).

To move to the left the patient rotates the left hip uppermost and the physiotherapist reverses her pressures.

For trunk flexion and movement to the right, the patient turns his pelvis so that the left hip is uppermost and the patient pulls his legs to the right.

This pattern can be adapted for patients who have stiff or painful

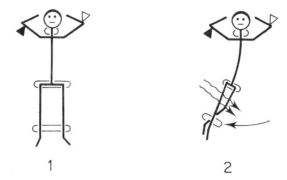

Fig. 7.11. Modification of trunk side-flexion pattern to gain trunk extension with rotation of the pelvis. 1) Starting position. 2) Right leg uppermost, pelvis rotates to the left.

shoulders by fixing on the scapula instead of the elbows so the arms are not in the neck rest position. When the patient moves to the right the physiotherapist places her right hand under the right scapula and pulls up while her left hand is placed over the left scapula and pushes down to give counter-resistance to the movement.

Trunk side-flexion pattern with upper trunk moving
The patient lies supine with a neck float while the physiotherapist stands between patient's legs and holds on the thighs (lateral aspects). The patient is commanded to bend his upper trunk to one side and at the same time the physiotherapist moves the patient to the same side. This movement can be performed slowly or quickly in a small or large range, but it is unlikely to be a large range movement done quickly. The slower the movement and the smaller the range, the easier the exercise. Other progressions can be made by making the body less streamlined. Initially the patient's arms are held in adduction and this is progressed by maintaining the arms in an abducted position and further progressed by holding bats in the hands (Fig. 7.12).

The physiotherapist can alter the difficulty of the exercise by altering the point of fixation. To make the pattern easier fixation is made at the pelvis but to make it harder fixation is moved distally to the lower legs or feet.

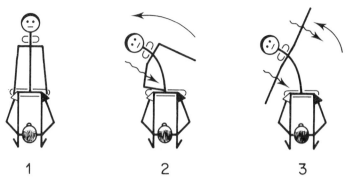

Fig. 7.12. Trunk side-flexion with upper trunk moving and the pelvis and legs fixed. 1) Starting position. 2) Patient side-flexes to right. Pelvis and legs steadied. 3) Progression with the arms in abduction. *N.B.* Pelvic float is optional.

Trunk flexion and extension patterns
The patient lies on his side turned 45° towards lying with the underneath arm out of the body ring and a neck float if desired (see Fig. 8.5). The physiotherapist stands in front of the patient and places her hands on opposite sides of the pelvis with the underneath hand slightly higher than the top hand.

For the flexor pattern the patient starts with the trunk in extension. The patient then flexes the trunk moving through the arc of a circle and rotating the upper trunk forwards from the uppermost shoulder. At the same time, the physiotherapist moves backwards moving the point of fixation. When full flexion has been achieved the patient relaxes and the physiotherapist stretches him out and the trunk is extended ready for the pattern to be repeated (Fig. 7.13).

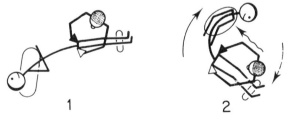

Fig. 7.13. Trunk flexion pattern. 1) Starting position. 2) Patient flexes trunk and at the same time the physiotherapist moves to her left, in a clockwise direction.

For the extensor pattern the patient is in side lying with his trunk flexed. He then extends his trunk with the uppermost shoulder and the head rotating backwards. At the same time, the physiotherapist moves forwards so that the point of fixation is moved, and as the body describes the arc of a circle through the water. When full extension has been achieved, the patient relaxes and the physiotherapist flexes the patient's trunk ready for the pattern to be repeated.

When handling children it is possible to hold firmly around the feet to work hips, knees and feet with the trunk. To attempt to do this with adults results in a very long lever making it virtually impossible for the physiotherapist to have control and give adequate fixation.

Trunk extension with rotation to the left and trunk flexion with rotation to the right

For these patterns the patient is in supine lying with the trunk flexed and rotated to the right with floats round the pelvis and neck while the physiotherapist stabilizes herself in walk, standing with the back foot against the side of the pool. She places her hands on the dorsal aspect of the patient's feet well below the surface of the water. The patient pushes away, extending his trunk and rotating his legs and trunk to the left. On completing that movement the patient then pulls himself towards the physiotherapist by flexing his trunk and legs and rotating to the right. Thus the physiotherapist remains still throughout both patterns (Fig. 7.14).

UPPER LIMB

Single-arm abduction pattern

The patient lies in supine supported by neck and pelvis floats and a small ring around both feet. The physiotherapist stands at the shoulder and places one hand over the dorsum of the patient's wrist and hand and the other hand over the lateral aspect of the patient's upper arm. The patient is instructed to push his body away from his arm, extending the wrist and fingers and laterally rotating the shoulder. He moves through the arc of a circle because the therapist provides fixation and leans into the movement as the patient moves away. At the end of the movement the patient relaxes, the therapist moves towards the patient and brings his arm to his side in

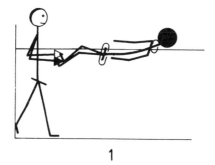

1

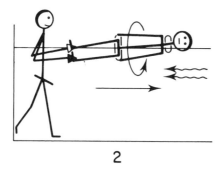

2

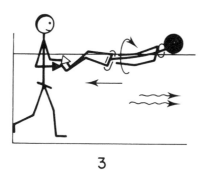

3

Fig. 7.14. Trunk extension with rotation to the left and trunk flexion with rotation to the right. 1) Starting position. 2) Patient extends trunk and rotates to left. 3) Patient flexes trunk and rotates to the right.

preparation for the pattern to be repeated (Fig. 7.15). Initially the resistance is great but towards the end of the movement momentum carries the patient's body away, forcing the shoulder into abduction and elevation. This is unsuitable for a painful shoulder joint. It can be avoided by the therapist either taking the fixation away by removing her hands from the patient or taking a short step forward before the painful range is reached.

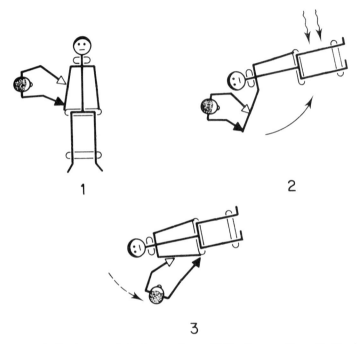

Fig. 7.15. Single-arm abduction pattern. 1) Starting position. 2) Physiotherapist plus patient's right arm are steady. Patient's body moves to left and right shoulder is abducted. 3) Physiotherapist walks towards patient adducting patient's right shoulder.

Single-arm adduction pattern

This is the reverse of the previous pattern. The patient lies in supine supported by floats, as for the abduction pattern, with the affected arm in elevation and lateral rotation and the elbow, wrist and fingers all extended. The manual hold of the physiotherapist is now changed with one hand on the flexor aspect of the hand and wrist and the other hand on the inner aspect of the upper arm. The patient is instructed to grip the physiotherapist's hand, flexing the wrist and fingers, pulling his trunk towards his arm and medially rotating at the shoulder. As the patient brings his trunk towards his arm the therapist moves the point of fixation (i.e. the arm) further away. Thus the patient describes an arc of a circle in the water. When the movement is completed the patient relaxes, the therapist moves back and returns his arm to the starting position in preparation for the pattern to be repeated (Fig. 7.16).

The therapist can increase the resistance for the patient by placing the proximal hand on the lateral border of the patient's

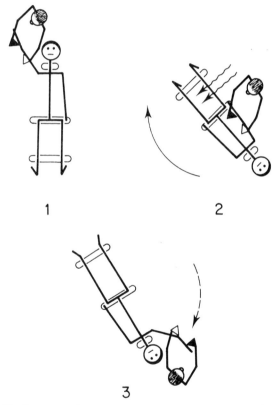

Fig. 7.16. Single-arm adduction. 1) Starting position. 2) Physiotherapist plus patient's right arm are steady. Patient's body moves to right and right shoulder is adducted. 3) Physiotherapist walks backwards and abducts patient's right shoulder.

scapula instead of his upper arm. The other hand can be placed anywhere on the patient's arm between the elbow and the fingers, such that the more distal this hand is the greater the effort demanded from the patient.

Bilateral flexion, abduction and lateral rotation
The patient lies supine supported by neck and pelvic floats with a small ring around both feet. The patient's arms are adducted with the elbows flexed and the therapist stands behind the patient's head. The palms of her hands are placed against the palms of the patient's hands. The movement begins by the patient pushing against the therapist's hands thus moving away from her by flexing, abducting and laterally rotating both arms. When the movement is complete the patient relaxes, the therapist takes the patient's arms back to the starting position by moving towards the patient, and the movement can be repeated (Fig. 7.17).

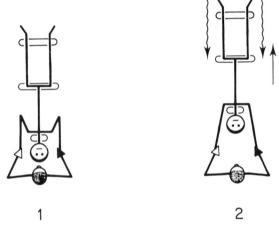

                    1   2

Fig. 7.17. Bilateral flexion, abduction and lateral rotation of the arms. 1) Starting position. 2) Elbows extend, shoulders are abducted, flexed and laterally rotated, the patient moves in the direction indicated.

Bilateral extension, adduction and medial rotation
The patient lies supine as in the previous pattern, and again the therapist stands behind the patient's head. For the starting position the patient's arms are flexed, abducted and laterally rotated and the grip is the same as with the previous pattern. The patient grips the

therapist's hands, then pulls his body towards the therapist by extending and adducting the shoulder while flexing the elbow. When the movement is complete the patient relaxes, the therapist moves back and takes the patient's arms into flexion, abduction and lateral rotation ready to repeat the pattern (Fig. 7.18).

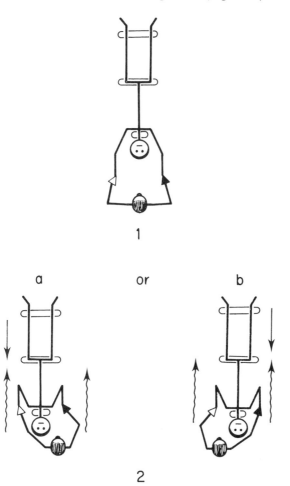

Fig. 7.18. Bilateral extension, adduction and medial rotation patterns of the arms. 1) Starting position. 2) Physiotherapist stands still, patient moves so that the elbows flex and the shoulders are extended, adducted and medially rotated. The patient may move to either side of the therapist, but it is usual to repeat to one side only, not to alternate.

Arm patterns in the prone position

For the following patterns the patient is lying prone with floats around the pelvis and feet. He may like a neck support but often patients prefer not to have a ring support at the neck when lying prone. In all the patterns the elbows are kept straight. The physiotherapist stands in front of the patient with her feet parallel to the pattern of movement.

For flexion, abduction and lateral rotation of the left shoulder the physiotherapist grasps the back of the patient's left hand with her right hand. The patient's arm is placed in extension, adduction and medial rotation and his head is over the therapist's right shoulder. The patient pushes his body away from the therapist as he flexes, abducts and laterally rotates the left shoulder, and extends the wrist and fingers. The physiotherapist's other hand is best used to guide the movement as she places it over the upper arm (Fig. 7.19). The

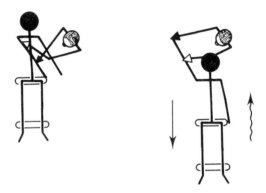

Fig. 7.19. Flexion, abduction and lateral rotation pattern. 1) Starting position with patient's arm in extension, adduction and medial rotation. 2) Patient flexes, abducts and laterally rotates left arm.

movement of the patient's arm is shown in Fig. 7.21. At the end of the movement, the patient relaxes and the physiotherapist steps forward to return the arm to the starting position.

For the extension, adduction and medial rotation of the left shoulder the patient's arm is placed in flexion, abduction and lateral rotation and his left hand grasps the physiotherapist's left hand.

The patient pulls his body towards the physiotherapist as he extends, adducts and medially rotates the left shoulder and flexes

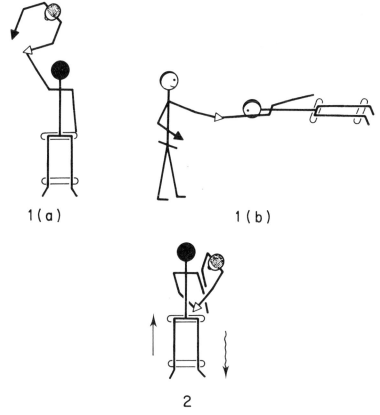

1 (a)

1 (b)

2

Fig. 7.20. Extension, adduction and medial rotation of the left arm. 1) a) Starting position. Patient's left arm in flexion, abduction and lateral rotation. b) Side view of starting position. 2) Patient extends, adducts and medially rotates left arm. The patient's head moves past the therapist's right shoulder.

the wrist and fingers. The physiotherapist's other hand may be placed over the inner aspect of the left upper arm.

As the movement is completed the patient moves over the therapist's right shoulder. On completion of the movement the patient relaxes, the therapist moves backwards and the patient's arm is returned to the starting position (Fig. 7.20).

The flexion, adduction (and lateral rotation pattern) and extension, abduction (and medial rotation) patterns are performed

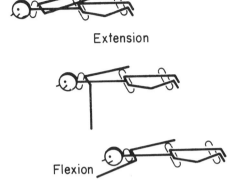

Extension

Flexion

Fig. 7.21. Illustration of patient's arm position in Figs 7.19 and 7.20.

in a similar way, but the patient moves away from or over the physiotherapist's left shoulder if the muscles of the left arm are working.

Some patients are nervous of lying prone in the water and these patterns should not be attempted with such patients on their first pool treatment sessions.

The opposite patterns can be performed one after the other so that the patient moves backwards and forwards over the same area, i.e. a flexor pattern follows an extensor pattern or an abduction pattern follows an adduction pattern. Each movement, however, must be completed as far as possible to be most effective. This technique is useful if the pool is small and it is not possible for the patient to move across the pool.

ISOMETRIC PATTERNS

In these patterns the patient is again supported in floats in the supine position and holds a position while the physiotherapist moves him in such a way that the turbulence and bow wave produced by the movement of the body in water resists the muscle contraction of the patient. This produces isometric contraction of the patient's muscles. The demand on the muscles will increase if the patient is moved quickly through the water by the physiotherapist because more turbulence is created. In a large pool the patient is moved in one direction, but in a small pool the patient is moved only short distances and the direction of movement is changed quickly from one to another.

Leg abduction pattern
The patient abducts both legs and the physiotherapists places her hands on the outer aspects of one thigh and lower leg. The patient is told to hold both legs apart and the physiotherapist pushes the patient round in a circle, working the abductors of the leg isometrically. For example, if the right leg is to be worked isometrically, the therapist's hands are applied to the left leg and the patient is moved by the therapist's walking in a clockwise direction (Fig. 7.22).

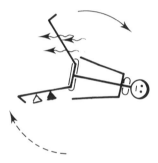

Fig. 7.22. Isometric work for the abductors of the leg. Right leg working isometrically.

Bilateral arm abduction
The patient lies with both arms abducted to 90° and the physiotherapist stands holding both feet. As the patient is pushed through the water he is told to keep both arms in the abducted position, thus working the abductors isometrically (Fig. 7.23).

For the adductors to work isometrically the patient keeps his arms in 45° of abduction and is pushed through the water by the physiotherapist, who stands at the patient's head.

Some of the basic patterns have been described, but the versatility of this method must be emphasized. The physiotherapist will find, as she becomes practised in the technique, the many ways in which it can be adapted to the individual patient's needs. Many patterns can be used with one limb stabilizing, that is, holding

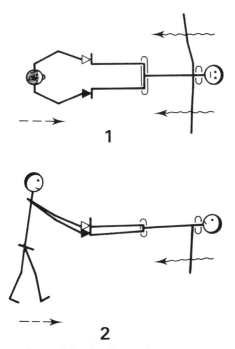

Fig. 7.23. Bilateral arm abduction isometric pattern. 1) Top view. 2) Side view.

isometrically whilst the other limb is working isotonically. For example, the lower-limb patterns may be applied with extension, abduction and medial rotation with the knee in extension held isometrically in one leg while the other leg works isotonically into flexion, adduction and lateral rotation with knee flexion. The physiotherapist's hands are placed on the patient's feet as for the basic patterns. At the end of the movement, the patient relaxes and the therapist extends the moving limbs passively. She will have to move slightly backwards, but not so far as when the isotonic pattern is used alone (Fig. 7.24). At first the pattern is repeated a few times with the same leg working isotonically, then the other leg is worked isotonically. Once the patient has learnt the patterns, coordination, in preparation for walking, may be improved by working the legs alternately isotonically and isometrically.

However, as in all hydrotherapy techniques, the therapist must be sure that the medium of water is being used to advantage and

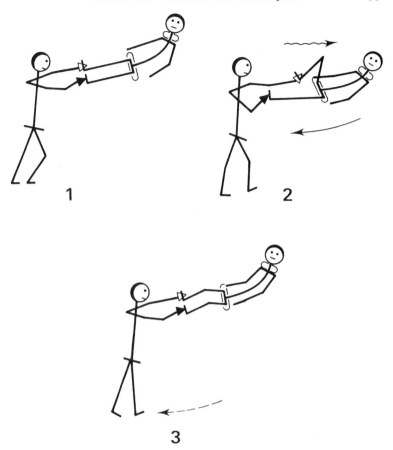

Fig. 7.24. Pattern working one limb isotonically and the other isometrically. 1) Starting position. 2) Patient flexes right leg. Left leg works isometrically. 3) Patient relaxes. Physiotherapist walks backwards and extends patient's left leg.

that she is not trying to use techniques in water which are better and more accurately done on dry land.

APPLICATION OF TECHNIQUES

Patients who are suitable for pool treatment fall into two broad categories:

1. those with joint problems in which there is usually diminished joint range, weakness of muscles with no neurological deficit and a varying degree of pain;
2. those with muscle weakness due to lower motor neurone pathology.

The use of Bad Ragaz techniques for patients with upper motor neurone deficit has not been found to be of value. It is felt that these patients, if handled in the medium of water, are better taught to swim, learning to develop the necessary balance, stability and movement by the use of head control and compensating for body asymmetry by moving various parts of the body around the datum point. The principles of this approach are in Chapter 11.

LIMITED RANGE OF MOTION, MUSCLE WEAKNESS AND PAIN
Patients presenting with these symptoms will be suffering from a variety of conditions, including osteoarthritis, rheumatoid arthritis and ankylosing spondylitis. They may have undergone orthopaedic surgery such as joint replacement, osteotomy or laminectomy, or they may require mobilization following fixation for fractures. Patients with these problems affecting the lower limbs and trunk benefit enormously from pool therapy and the techniques described above allow for careful and controlled handling of the patient.

In treating any disability of the lower limb it is essential to work for a strong and mobile trunk. Without this the patient will be severely hindered in all activities, however much recovery or improvement he obtains in the legs. Also, if treatment sessions are started working a part of the body away from the painful weak area, by overflow from the stronger less affected area, the weaker parts are more in a state of preparedness for activity.

On the patient's first pool session, as soon as he enters the water, a body ring and neck collar are put on. The patient lies supine, the physiotherapist supporting him proximally, i.e. around the scapular region or at the pelvis. By the manual holds the physiotherapist is able to have maximum control of the patient and prevent any rolling or instability occurring if the patient is not used to water.

Trunk-side flexion in supine should be given first, the physiotherapist's grip being adapted if the patient is very nervous. Instead of holding the patient's elbows she holds at the thorax in the scapula region, still giving the counter pressure with her hands as the patient moves his legs from side to side. Alternatively she can hold the pelvis and have the patient work from a fixed lower trunk. This is useful if the patient has pain and stiffness in the lower trunk and hips; in later treatments fixation can be given at the upper trunk or arms.

The patient can be turned into the side lying position and trunk flexion and extension patterns can be given, again with the physiotherapist holding proximally at the pelvis in the early treatments.

The unaffected or least-affected limb is then worked through as full a range as possible against maximal resistance in the single-leg flexion–extension and abduction–adduction patterns. The affected leg is worked firstly in the flexion–extension patterns. The physiotherapist has both of her hands on this extremity and can control, guide, resist or assist the movement as necessary. If the hip is the most painful joint, the physiotherapist can have both hands on the thigh; it is not always necessary or desirable to hold as distally as the foot. Abduction and adduction are best done using the bilateral patterns.

Patients needing trunk strengthening and mobilizing, for instance after laminectomy, are treated with strong single-leg and bilateral leg patterns followed by specific trunk patterns. Fixation should be proximal if there is a lot of pain and limitation of movement. Later treatments can include trunk flexion and extension in side lying with hip and knee movement, i.e. with more distal holds to work more of the body maximally.

Pool treatment is sometimes used for patients with pain and limitation of movement in the shoulder following fractures of the humerus, dislocation or frozen shoulders of unknown aetiology. The same principles of treatment apply as with the lower limb. Upper-trunk exercise precedes maximal work of the unaffected arm and is followed by movement patterns, at first in supine and later in prone, to strengthen and mobilize the affected shoulder.

MUSCLE WEAKNESS WITH LOWER MOTOR NEURONE PATHOLOGY

Patients in this group can be treated to great advantage in the water and by these techniques, not least because of the ease of handling the severely handicapped. In these cases pain is seldom a main problem and maximal work through full range can be given to all muscles, whether they be grade 1 or grade 4.

The strongest parts must be worked first so that use can be made of overflow. Bilateral leg patterns are very useful when one leg is stronger than the other; again overflow is used. In strengthening exercises, the speed, length of lever and rate of change of direction all can be used to increase resistance, using turbulence and wave formation. The stronger the work required, so must the physiotherapist fix more firmly. It is most important that her stance and her body weight are used efficiently, thus allowing for economy of effort whilst still obtaining the maximum work from the patient.

SWIMMING

This is an excellent recreational activity that facilitates coordination, provides strong muscle work and a large range of joint movement for the whole body, and is valuable for almost every patient. Various swimming strokes can be used to exercise particular muscles and joints. In both breast stroke and back stroke the hip joint is abducted and laterally rotated; therefore the muscles should be sufficiently strong to guard the joint before allowing these strokes to be performed. In breast stroke the arm movements involve elevation of the shoulder followed by medial rotation and extension of the shoulder joint and retraction of the scapula. The crawl (freestyle) stroke entails strong muscle work for the extensor muscles of the hip and back. In the front crawl the arms are strongly adducted and extended, while in the back crawl they are flexed, elevated and abducted.

Swimming is taught using the Halliwick principles described in Chapter 11. Every handicapped person has a different balance difficulty and each one is taught to float on his back without any flotation equipment. Initially this is carried out on a one-to-one ratio of therapist (instructor) to patient. Before the therapist allows the patient independence, breathing control and safety and recovery are taught (see Chapter 11). The patient must learn to breathe out if the head is under the water and taught to regain a safe position on his back by turning the head and rotating forwards or sideways. Once the patient can float and control his body in the supine position, movement of the body is produced passively by the therapist creating turbulence at the head or under the patient's thorax. The therapist stands at the patient's head, walks backwards and the patient 'glides' along. This method is good in the presence of spasticity because the therapist avoids touching the patient, thereby reducing the risk of increasing the spasticity. Further progression in swimming is achieved by teaching the patient a sculling action in which he starts to base movement on the balanced floating position. He is instructed to move his hands slowly from side to side, keeping the palms down and the fingers extended, at the level of the pelvis, which is near the body's centre of gravity. This allows the patient to move independently, the faster and more continuous the sculling action the quicker the patient progresses through the water. Eventually the swimmer will bring both arms out of the water as in a back crawl action. Some patients will be able to progress to swimming on the side and prone.

Breast stroke is useful for mobilizing all limb movements and improving coordination; the crawl aids thoracic and shoulder mobility and strengthens limb muscles; the butterfly stroke strengthens muscles and mobilizes joints of the upper limb in addition to mobilizing the spine; the side stroke mobilizes the lower limb joints and thorax.

RE-EDUCATION IN WALKING

The following will act as a guideline where walking re-education is required.

The patient stands within parallel bars, or if these are not available a walking frame may be used. The physiotherapist stands in front of the patient and supports him at the pelvis if necessary. The following movements are performed:

1. weight transference from side to side;
2. weight transference forwards and backwards;
3. walking forwards.

As the patient walks the hands are moved along the bars as they would if he were using crutches or sticks, that is in the same order and the same distance apart.

The physiotherapist corrects any abnormal pattern in the gait, such as not pushing off properly or bending the knee to carry the leg forward. She must also ensure that the patient leans slightly forwards, because due to the build up of pressure in front there is a tendency for the body weight to remain back on the heels and with the upthrust of buoyancy he is inclined to overbalance backwards.

To progress, the patient moves out of the parallel bars but the physiotherapist still remains in front of the patient supporting him at the pelvis or shoulders (see Fig. 10.5, p. 170). The patient rests his hands on her shoulders and the exercises above are repeated. The faster the patient walks, the greater the 'wake' made by the physiotherapist in front who is walking backwards and therefore the easier it is for the patient. For further progression the patient holds a large float instead of being supported by the physiotherapist, who moves from the front to the side of the patient so that he then walks unassisted. The physiotherapist then walks behind the patient, in his wake, so as to increase the drag effect and provide resistance. Muscle power can be further strengthened in the later stages by resisted walking. For this the physiotherapist stands behind the patient applying manual resistance at the pelvis.

In carrying the leg forward buoyancy assists both the push off by the calf muscles and hip and knee flexion, but the hip extensors have to work against buoyancy in lowering the leg. This muscle work is different from that of walking on land.

When the patient can walk well in the pool, re-education should continue on land to ensure that the patient adjusts his walking pattern to his normal environment.

8

Treatment of Rheumatic Disorders

CLINICAL SIGNS AND SYMPTOMS

Pain in and around the affected joints leads to tension and spasm in certain muscle groups acting on them. In the pool, the warmth of the water surrounding the joint relieves pain and helps relaxation and so brings further relief of pain. The buoyancy of the water decreases the strain on joints.

Limitation of movement and stiffness in joints is decreased, partly owing to the relief of pain and partly owing to the support of buoyancy during movement.

Muscle weakness in groups surrounding the part can be improved by graduated excercises. At first buoyancy is used to assist the muscle. Gradually the effect of buoyancy is diminished until the exercises can be performed using buoyancy as a resistance.

Deformity is a characteristic of certain conditions. Again the warmth of the water helps the muscles to relax, and as a result further correction of the deformity can be achieved.

Functional ability is improved as the exercises help to improve muscle function, thus building up the patient's confidence in his ability to perform similar movements on land.

RHEUMATOID ARTHRITIS (RA)

Rheumatoid arthritis is a non-suppurative, inflammatory polyarthritis characteristically involving peripheral joints, often symmetrically, and running a subacute to chronic course of exacerbations and remissions. Weight loss and slight fever, and also extra-articular features involving connective tissue and other organs, often occur. It is a generalized condition affecting a number of joints; therefore a patient may have some joints at a painful stage and some pain-free.

Hydrotherapy is recommended when the disease is subacute, whilst the patient is still on bed rest following a period of complete rest, or in the chronic stage. Patients whose symptoms worsen in damp weather may not be suitable for hydrotherapy.

Treatment during an acute exacerbation is contraindicated, but a patient with one acute joint may be treated in the pool with the affected joint protected in a plastazote splint.

A plastazote collar may be worn if the patient has severe changes in the cervical spine. If a knee joint is unstable or painful, or both, a plastazote splint or polythene reinforcement is helpful, especially whilst the patient is lifted in and out of the pool.

The main contraindication, apart from general contraindications, is that in the very early stage of recovery from an acute generalized episode of RA the necessary dressing and undressing may be too tiring.

AIMS OF TREATMENT
1. Relief of pain and muscle spasm
2. Maintenance or restoration of muscle power around painful joints
3. Reduction of deformity and increase of range of movement in all affected joints.
4. Maintenance of range of movement and muscle power of unaffected joints.
5. Restoration of confidence and re-education of function.

TECHNIQUES
Since rheumatoid patients tire quickly, the pool therapy programme must be devised to take this into account. For the first treatment session, 10 minutes may be long enough. Then at subsequent sessions the time in the water may be increased to 15 or 20 minutes.

The number of exercises and repetitions must also be gauged according to each individual's ability.

Head support lying is a good starting position for initial treatments because the physiotherapist has control over the patient's limbs, trunk and neck. In float support lying, patients may flex the neck to avoid water entering the ears or the hair getting wet.

Relaxation
The patient enters, or is lifted slowly and carefully into, the water and is familiarized with the size and the depth of the pool and the equipment. The patient is then introduced to the supporting effect of buoyancy in H sup. ly; or fl. sup. ly. The contrast method of relaxation and breathing exercises can be very helpful. If the patient is very nervous, sitting may be a more suitable starting position.

Mobilization
For painful joints this is carried out with active assisted movements, active sweeping movements counteracting deformity or pattern movements, as in techniques developed at Bad Ragaz (Chapter 7). Movement of any very painful or acute joints must be avoided, but as pain and swelling subside assisted active movements should be added.

Strengthening
Strengthening of muscles surrounding a painful joint can be achieved by isometric contractions or stabilizations (Fig. 8.1).

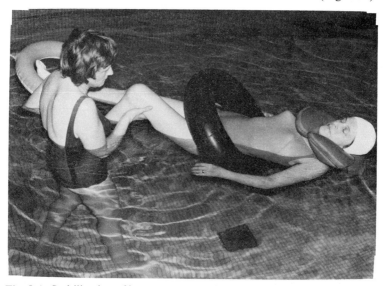

Fig. 8.1. Stabilization of knee, co-contraction of muscle groups around the joint.

Isometric contractions can be achieved by the patient trying to push against a very large float much less dense than water, or by the patient being asked to 'hold' a position while being pushed through the water by the therapist (see Chapter 7).

For strengthening muscles around pain-free joints, use is made of finely graded exercises by using buoyancy, altering speed of movement or length of weight-arm, creating turbulence, using equipment and using patterns of movement. The patterns chosen are those which move pain-free joints and counteract the deformity produced by the disease, e.g. abduction with lateral rotation of the shoulder (Fig. 8.2).

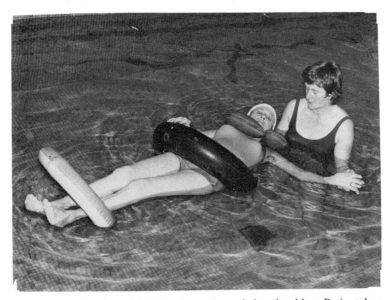

Fig. 8.2. Abduction with lateral rotation of the shoulder. Patient has limitation of joint range with pain. The therapist is able, with her hands, to control the movement with accuracy.

When the patient moves away from the therapist, the free movement stops only when the limit of joint range is reached, whether this is normal or restricted by contractures or muscle spasm. Momentum often tends to carry the patient beyond this point. In a normal joint this effect does not matter, but in RA uncontrolled stretching is contraindicated. The technique is modified to prevent this stretching effect which could damage periarticular structures and initiate or increase the inflammatory process.

This modification is achieved by (a) holding the scapula with one hand, instead of having both hands on the patient's upper limb; (b) removing the distal hand, thus removing counterpressure, so that the movement stops; and (c) the therapist taking short steps forward just before the limit of the range is reached.

Other modifications which may be necessary. In using the trunk side-flexion pattern, the neck-rest position might not be possible if the upper limbs are affected and the therapist must fix the patient on the scapulae as described in Chapter 7 (Fig. 8.3).

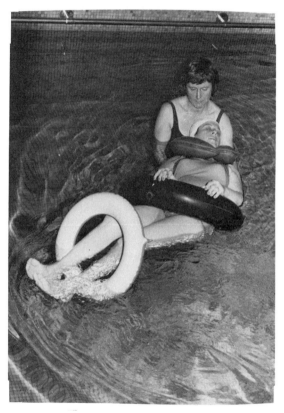

Fig. 8.3. Trunk side-flexion pattern, showing modified starting position with fixation on the scapulae.

Any starting position which requires an overhead grip, with the patient in the floating position, is contraindicated.

In some abduction patterns of the lower limbs there may be a strain on the knee joint if the resistance is given through the lateral aspect of the foot or ankle. In RA with knee involvement this may be better avoided or adapted so that the therapist applies counter pressure and support on the lateral aspect of the knee.

A correcting element of posture and function should always be present during the treatment.

Walking

In RA, patients may have a dorsiflexion and eversion deformity of the foot, resulting in a valgus position and no 'push off' during walking. This movement is much easier in the pool and should be re-educated there before attempting it on land.

Swimming

Breast stroke is suitable if joints in the upper limbs are pain-free and no, or minimal, changes in the cervical spine are present. Otherwise back stroke, with arm movements within the pain-free limit, can be taught. The thrust in the lower limb is provided by hip and knee extension with plantar flexion.

EARLY EXERCISES

The following patterns and exercises are a guide to treatment, but must, of course, be modified to suit individual patients.

1. H sup. ly; deep-breathing exercises, general tensing followed by relaxation.
2. ½ sup. ly; (float at F)—alt. Toe and Ank bend and stretch.
3. ½ sup. ly; (float at F)—alt. Hip and K bend and stretch.
4. ½ sup. ly; (float at F)—L part and close.
5. ½ sup. ly; (float at F)—L turn in and out.
6. bd. sitt; (strap around Thigh)—Fing, Wrist and Elb. stretch f. and bend.
7. bd sitt; (strap around Thigh)—Fing, Wrist and Elb. stretch s. and bend.
8. H sup. ly; A carry s. and u. and lower.
9. H sup. ly; Hnd, turn u. and d.

10. walking round the pool, stressing Hip and K bending and stretching.
11. sitt; Stand u. (with push from F).

STRONGER EXERCISES
12. rch. gr. st; 1Hip and K bend and stretch.
13. ½ yd. gr. st; 1L carry f. and b.
14. sitt; alt. K stretch and bend (with F movements).
15. sitt; A carry f., s. and d.
16. sitt; A raise s. and press d.
17. bd. sitt; T turn from s. to s.
18. yd. sitt; T turn from s. to s.
19. ½ sup. ly; A carry o. to yd. and return.
20. ½ sup: s: ly; (float at F)—Hip and K bend and stretch to full extension.
21. ½ sup. ly; (float at F)—1L push d. and raise slowly.
22. fl. sup. ly; L press d. and raise slowly.
23. walk sidewards, backwards and climb stairs.

Progression. Add streamlined, then unstreamlined, bats to exercises 7, 8, 15, 16, 18 and 19.

PATTERNS OF MOVEMENT
1. Abduction and external rotation of the shoulder.
2. Extension, abduction and medial rotation of the hip.
3. Bilateral abduction of the lower limbs (note that care is required if the knee joints are affected).
4. Trunk side-flexion with lower trunk, pelvis and legs moving.
5. Trunk side-flexion with upper trunk moving.
6. Isometric patterns, with abduction and lateral rotation of the arms and abduction of the legs.

POLYMYALGIA RHEUMATICA

Patients nearly always suffer from pain, weakness and morning stiffness in the muscles around the neck, shoulders, back and thighs, with absence of joint swelling and reduction of movement. If applied sensitively, hydrotherapy can be very helpful in reducing pain, maintaining muscle power and range of movement, and in boosting the patients' confidence. These patients may not need more than six to eight sessions in the pool. The duration of the initial session is short and gradually increased from session to session. If signs of fatigue are observed the treatment should be interrupted and the patient should rest.

For strengthening, sweeping movements should be carried out, using buoyancy to support and assist at first. There should then be a progression against buoyancy, and adding floats or altering the lever arm.

Isotonic arm, leg and trunk patterns of the Bad Ragaz technique can be useful.

Swimming helps to improve patients' endurance and power and restores morale.

ANKYLOSING SPONDYLITIS (AS)

This is a sero-negative inflammatory arthropathy affecting the sacroiliac joints, the spinal and thoracic joints and sometimes the hip and shoulder joints. It is more common in men than in women, usually affecting the 20–40 age group.

Early recognition and good management—not least on the part of the patient—have reduced the likelihood of the severe deformity and rigidity which used to characterize the condition.

Hydrotherapy plays an important part in the treatment of patients with ankylosing spondylitis. Pool treatment is usually given in conjunction with exercise sessions on land, where back care and home exercises are taught. Patients may need to repeat a course of exercises once or twice a year and they are encouraged to take up swimming and join a swimming club.

During examination and assessment of a patient with AS it is particularly important to measure thoracic expansion and vital capacity. Patients with a vital capacity below 1 litre may be treated in the pool but require close supervision. Sometimes it may be necessary to treat patients on land first and add pool treatment when the vital capacity has increased.

Patients with AS should enter the pool slowly to get accustomed to the effect of hydrostatic pressure on the thorax, and starting positions first chosen may have the thorax out of the water, e.g. $\frac{1}{2}$ sup. ly; or sitting on a high stool (or the pool steps).

Patients with AS will come for pool treatment at various stages of the disease, so the principles of treatment must vary accordingly.

AIMS OF TREATMENT
A. *During initial recovery from an acute phase*
   1. Reduction of pain and muscle spasm in the neck, shoulder girdle, thoracic and lumbar spines, and, if necessary, the hips.
   2. Improvement of respiratory expansion, increase of vital capacity and correction of the patient's breathing pattern.
   3. Maintenance of mobility of the hip and shoulder joints.

B. *When pain and muscle spasm have decreased*
   1. Mobilization of the thoracic and lumbar spines.
   2. Correction of posture.
   3. Restoration of muscle balance, especially in the trunk muscles.
   4. Teaching swimming.

C. *Final rehabilitation*
   1. Strengthening of the extensor muscles to counteract the flexion deformity.
   2. Improvement of the respiratory function and swimming activities.

TECHNIQUES
It is worth noting that the patients are often younger men and the strengthening exercises can therefore be stronger than those given to patients with other rheumatic diseases.

For the first two or three sessions in the pool the main theme is relaxation, for which the starting position of choice is fl. sup. ly. The therapist stands between the patient's ankles, fixing both knees, and the patient is then moved passively from side to side, with large sweeping movements, while the therapist walks backwards. The patient is asked to release the tension in neck and shoulders and let the movement 'happen'. It may be helpful to teach the patient the contrast relaxation method prior to this exercise, either on land or in the water in ½ sup. ly; or fl. sup. ly.

Once the patient is able to relax, he can be asked to join in and follow the movement actively, letting the momentum of the movement of the body gain range of movement.

The therapist can also stand behind the patient's head, fix on the pelvis and move the patient in a similar manner so that the legs swing freely. As the patient improves, the therapist's fixation may be altered so that the lumbar and then thoracic spines may begin to move.

These principles can be applied to other trunk patterns. More trunk side-flexion and rotation can also be achieved by the breathing exercises described in Chapter 6 (Fig. 8.4).

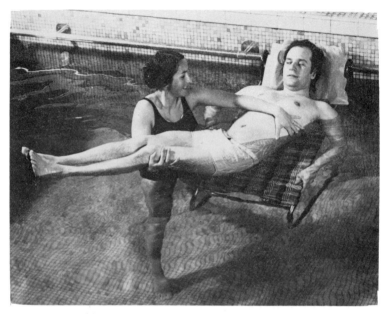

Fig. 8.4. Breathing exercises with trunk side-flexion to gain expansion of left lung.

The hold–relax technique can be used to increase hip extension— $\frac{1}{2}$ sup. pr. ly; hold 1L d. and let it come up.

To increase shoulder abduction—fl. ly; (bat in right Hnd)—right A is carried o. to yd.; the therapist holds the patient's pelvis and moves the patient in a circle to his right. During this movement the patient 'holds' the arm and then releases carefully. For neck extension—fl. sup. ly; (floats at F); the therapist's hands are underneath the patient's head, the patient pushes the head back into her hands and 'holds'. while the therapist walks backwards, and then releases slowly.

For strengthening, use is made of buoyancy, increased lever arm, increased speed and turbulence, floats, rings and bats. Repeated contractions can be used to strengthen the back extensor muscles, the abdominals and hip abduction, rotation and extension. All Bad Ragaz movement patterns (Chapter 7) of the arms, legs and trunk can be applied, starting with arms and legs, then progressing to the trunk. On the whole, trunk flexion patterns are best avoided.

Swimming
The patient should learn to float (without supporting ring or floats) and to swim on his back using the Halliwick principles (Chapter 11). Only when the cervical and thoracic spine extend sufficiently should the patient be taught breast stroke and front crawl. The patient can then improve his breathing control, by holding his breath under water and slowly exhaling into the water. He can then increase the number of strokes to each breath, and finally swim under water.

EARLY EXERCISES
1. sitt; Breathing exercises; progress by sitting in deeper water.
2. $\frac{1}{2}$ sup. ly; (or fl. sup. ly;)—deep br. exs and relaxation by contrast method.
3. $\frac{1}{2}$ sup. ly; (float on F)—L part and close.
4. $\frac{1}{2}$ sup. ly; (float on F)—Hip and K bend and stretch.
5. $\frac{1}{2}$ sup. s. ly; 1 Hip and K bend f. and stretch b. to full ext.
6. $\frac{1}{2}$ sup. s. ly; Hip and K bend and stretch.
7. $\frac{1}{2}$ sup. ly; 1L press d. and return.
8. $\frac{1}{2}$ sup. ly; L press d. and return.
9. sitt; A raise to yd. and return.
10. sitt; A to rch, to yd. and press down (avoid protraction of shoulder).
11. sitt; Sh. girdle push b. and return (retract shoulder).

Appropriate patterns
Bilateral hip extension, abduction and medial rotation.
Bilateral arm patterns.
Arm abduction and lateral rotation.
Arm adduction and medial rotation.

INTERMEDIATE EXERCISES
12. Rch. sitt; T turn s. to s.
13. sitt; Hollow and hump lower back.
14. Toe sup. ly; T, Hip and K bend and stretch.

15. Toe sup. ly; T bend s.
16. ½ sup. ly; Breast stroke leg action.
17. ½ sup. ly; Back crawl leg action.
18. ½ sup. ly; H and F press back followed by relaxation.
19. ½ sup. pr. ly; T, Hip and K bend and stretch.
20. ½ sup. pr. ly; Inspiration with H turn to s., expiration with H turn forward into water (as in swimming).
21. fl. sup. ly; A carry s. and return.
22. fl. sup. ly; A push d. and raise slowly.
23. Walking backwards through pool.

APPROPRIATE PATTERNS
Trunk extension in side lying (Fig. 8.5).
Trunk side-flexion with extension with lower trunk, pelvis, and legs moving.

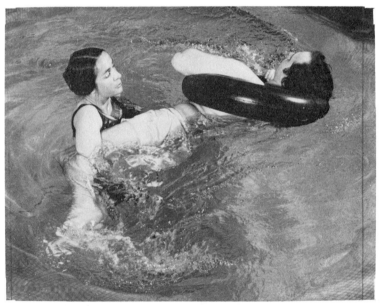

Fig. 8.5. Trunk extension pattern.

ADVANCED EXERCISES
24. yd. Toe sup. ly; T bend s. to s.
25. yd. Toe sup. ly; T Hip and K bend and stretch.

26. ½ sup. pr. ly; Breast stroke leg action.
27. fl. sup. ly; H press b. and relax.
28. fl. sup. ly; A and L push b. and relax.
29. fl. sup. ly; H, A and L push b. and relax.
30. gr. st. (parallel bars); L and T stretch b. and return (with Hip & K bending).

Progression. Progress by adding floats or flippers and adding bats, which may then be changed from streamlined to unstreamlined (Fig. 8.6).

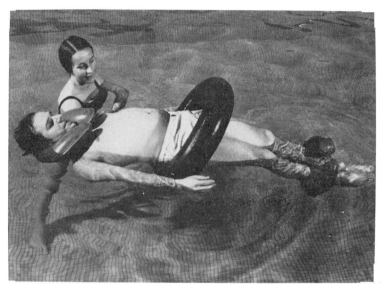

Fig. 8.6. Back extension against buoyancy and floats.

Appropriate patterns
Patterns are progressed from the intermediate stage by increasing the number of repetitions, making the body more unstreamlined and moving the point of fixation.

JUVENILE CHRONIC POLYARTHRITIS

This term covers rheumatoid arthritis, ankylosing spondylitis, polyarticular disease and psoriatic arthritis in children, i.e. up to the age of 16.

Water is an excellent medium for treating children with these arthropathies, because there are therapeutic, recreational, psychological and social benefits with no clear demarcation between therapy and play.

Children may be treated individually or in groups. There are advantages in group therapy because it is possible to increase the variety of games and activities, thereby achieving more enjoyment and social interaction for each child. They feel happy in the pool, work hard and subconsciously move their joints through a greater range of movement. Water may be used as a medium to facilitate extension movements to counteract the flexion deformities characteristic of juvenile arthritis. Movement from the vertical to the horizontal position encourages extension movements of the head followed by the rest of the body.

The 'stick' position (Fig. 11.2) is unstable and must be taught to control the body.

When a child has mastered body control in the horizontal position he is taught to move in this position. Breathing control must be taught to ensure that the child is safe in water, and to improve chest expansion and respiratory function.

Once a child has control both of breathing and of body movement in the horizontal position, swimming may be taught.

Activities such as kangaroo jumps will encourage extension of the hips and knees. The child rests his hands on the therapist's forearms or hands and jumps across the pool. On each jump, he is encouraged to extend the legs, and as he returns to blow out when he reaches the water. The knee and hip extensors may also be strengthened by pushing floats down into the water.

OSTEOARTHRITIS (OA)

Patients with degenerative changes of the spinal, hip and knee joints are frequently recommended for hydrotherapy. Degenerative changes in one joint will cause an imbalance of other joints and muscles. In osteoarthritis of the hip joint, apparent shortening of one leg may develop (due to a flexion, adduction and lateral rotation deformity), and there may well be a compensatory lumbar scoliosis; or with a fixed flexion deformity of one or both hips the lumbar spine will compensate for this lack of extension by lumbar lordosis.

Hydrotherapy is particularly useful for patients with bilateral osteoarthritis of the hip or knee joints because of the weight relief provided by buoyancy. Patients may be treated in the early stages of the disease, whilst awaiting surgery, or occasionally after surgery.

Exercises are graded by taking advantage of the three uses of buoyancy, i.e. by assisting the movement, by supporting the limb to allow free movement, and finally by resisting the movement. By adding floats at the ankle (or a 'flipper') exercises can be made more strenuous.

Float support lying is often used as a starting position to promote relaxation, which will help to overcome localized muscle spasm around a stiff joint.

Reach grasp standing position is used when the force of buoyancy is required to assist flexion of the hip and knee or abduction of the hip.

It is to the patient's lasting benefit if he can learn to swim, or take up this pastime again. On completion of his course of treatment he can continue with the swimming and exercises at a public swimming bath, as this is an excellent way of maintaining his mobility and muscle strength.

AIMS OF TREATMENT FOR HIP OSTEOARTHRITIS
1. Relief of pain.
2. Relief of muscle spasm, especially in the hip flexors, adductors and lateral rotators.
3. Strengthening of all the muscles round the hip joint, with special emphasis on the extensors, abductors and medial rotators.
4. Mobilization of other joints, e.g. lumbar spine or knees.
5. Increase of range of movement of the affected joint, especially flexion, extension, abduction and medial rotation.
6. Improvement of walking pattern.
7. Teaching swimming.

TECHNIQUES (HIP OA)

Relaxation
The patient is supported in H sup. ly. or fl. sup. ly; and instructed in conscious relaxation. Then the therapist stands behind the patient's head, fixes on the pelvis and moves the patient from side to side with

large sweeping movements. Together with the warmth of the water, these techniques help relieve pain and reduce muscle spasm.

Mobilization
The hold–relax technique is used to gain relaxation of the muscles in spasm and thereby gain range of movement. For hip extension, the patient should be in ½ sup. incl. pr. st; so that buoyancy will help to gain the new movement. For hip abduction, the starting position may be ½ sup. s. ly; where the movement is very limited, and then progressed to ½ gr. incl. tow side st;.

Longitudinal oscillatory movements applied in the long axis of the femur with the hip in adduction help to gain range. The technique requires two physiotherapists, one to fix the pelvis and the other to apply the oscillatory technique (Fig. 8.7).

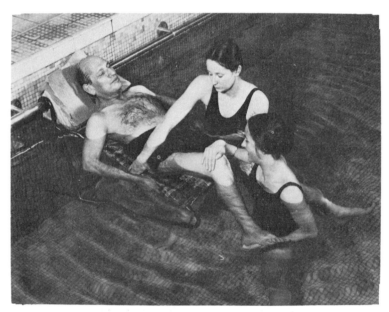

Fig. 8.7. Mobilizations to the right hip joint.

EXERCISES (HIP OA)
A selection of the following exercises is useful:
　1. ½ sup. ly; (K at rt L) F part. and clos. (keeping K tog. for Hip medial rotation).

2. $\frac{1}{2}$ sup. s. ly; 1 Hip and K bend and stretch.
3. $\frac{1}{2}$ sup. s. ly; bicycling action w. top L.
4. $\frac{1}{2}$ sup. pr. ly; K bend up (under stretcher) and stretch b.
5. $\frac{1}{2}$ sup. ly; L part and close.
6. $\frac{1}{2}$ sup. pr. ly; 1L raise and lower.
7. $\frac{1}{2}$ sup. s. ly; 1L raise s. and push d.
8. $\frac{1}{2}$ gr. incl. tow s. st; 1L raise and lower.
9. sitt; st. u. and sit d.
10. gr. incl. pr. st; 1L raise and lower.

All these exercises should be performed with slow sweeping movements.

Exercises suitable for strengthening
11. $\frac{1}{2}$ sup. ly; 1L press d. (w. flipper or float).
12. $\frac{1}{2}$ sup. s. ly; 1L press d. (w. flipper or float).
13. $\frac{1}{2}$ sup. s. ly; (K at rt L) lower leg push d. (for medial rotators).
14. gr. st; 1 Hip and K bend u. and push d. (add float).
15. $\frac{1}{2}$ sup. ly; alt L push u. and d. quickly (add flippers).
16. walking backwards.

Walking pattern
It is important that the therapist analyses the cause of any abnormality, e.g. pain, weakness of abductors leading to Trendelenburg gait or fixed flexion deformity producing a short-leg effect. Walking re-education will follow the method indicated in Chapter 6, with emphasis on hip extension of the weight-bearing limb during its stance phase. Instructions to the patient to keep the feet apart sideways is also usually required.

Swimming
The breast stroke is useful for gaining hip extension and abduction and the leg action may be performed as a separate exercise. The back crawl leg action will also help to strengthen the hip extensors.

PATTERNS OF MOVEMENT (HIP OA)
1. Bilateral extension–abduction pattern of the leg (Fig. 8.8).
2. Extension abduction and medial rotation of the hip, with knee extension.
3. Unilateral abduction with one leg working isotonically and the other working isometrically.

These patterns should be performed slowly to ensure full range and minimum turbulence.

Mobilizing for the unaffected joints is achieved by free active exercises and trunk patterns.

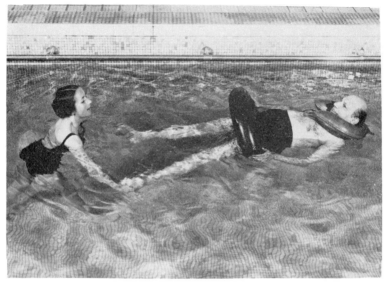

Fig. 8.8. Bilateral hip abduction pattern showing end of movement.

Strengthening

Where pain is a dominant feature, the muscles round the joint should be worked isometrically. This may be achieved by using isometric patterns, rhythmic stabilizations or large floats.

Useful patterns are: single-leg abduction pattern with the painful hip working isometrically or with the patient in std. fl. ly; and pushed through the water head first; or with the patient in fl. s. ly; with the therapist fixing the pelvis and swinging the legs backwards through the water while the patient holds into extension.

Rhythmic stabilizations are given with the patient in fl. ly;. If a large float is placed on the foot and the patient attempts to push the leg into the water in fl. ly. or ½ sup. ly. the muscles will work isometrically.

As movement becomes less painful muscles are worked isotonically, initially in a small range. For example, in fl. ly; with a ring round both ankles, the patient is asked to push both legs sideways or one leg downwards.

Patterns which are used for mobilizing are adopted for strengthening by increasing speed (to create turbulence) or by applying reversals.

For patients awaiting surgery, the emphasis should be on gaining mobility of the other hip, lumbar spine and knees and on strengthening the muscles of the affected hip.

Patients requiring hydrotherapy after surgery usually have a delayed recovery period because of a postoperative complication and the main difficulty is lack of joint movement. These patients usually respond to a programme of mobilization as indicated in the early stages. Pain is not usually a dominant feature and the programme can be fairly vigorous.

AIMS OF TREATMENT FOR KNEE OSTEOARTHRITIS
1. Relief of pain.
2. Relief of spasm of the hamstrings.
3. Increase of movement—often the last few degrees of extension.
4. Increase of strength of the quadriceps and, if necessary, the hamstrings and calf muscles.
5. Improvement of gait.
6. Maintenance of mobility of hips and ankles.

TECHNIQUES (KNEE OA)
Relaxation in float lying as for OA hip treatment. Hold–relax may be used to gain knee extension given in ½ sup. ly. or sitt.

EXERCISES (KNEE OA)
1. sitt.; K straighten and bend.
2. gr. st.; 1 Hip and K bend and stretch.
3. ½ sup. s. ly.; 1 Hip and K bend and stretch.
4. ½ sup. ly. (float under 1K)—quads contr.
5. gr. ½st.; 1K bend and stretch.
6. walking round pool, emphasising straight knee on stance phase.
7. gr. st.; alt K bend and stretch.
8. walking backwards.

9. sitt.; st. u. and sitt. d.
10. gr. st. (float on foot); 1 Hip and K bend and stretch d.

PATTERNS OF MOVEMENT (KNEE OA)
Suitable patterns are those incorporating knee movements applied with the same principles as for OA hip treatment.

9
Treatment of Neurological Disorders

Pool therapy is used in the treatment of many neurological disorders. The warmth and support of the water help to relieve some of the patient's symptoms, and a graduated progression of exercises is of value to patients whose muscles are weak or paralysed. As well as giving the patient support and freedom of movement, the warm water enables the physiotherapist to move him more easily than on land. As with other conditions, these factors improve both the patient's confidence and his morale.

CLINICAL SIGNS AND SYMPTOMS

Weakness or paralysis. A patient is said to be paralysed if he is unable to perform voluntary movement. When the upper motor neurone is affected, the patient is unable to initiate the voluntary movement, though the muscles remain capable of contracting. The condition is known as paralysis of movement. If the lower motor neurone is affected, the patient is unable to perform voluntary movement because the final common pathway is damaged and the ability of the muscles to contract is lost; this is known as paralysis of muscle. Lack of use leads eventually to muscle atrophy, which will hamper recovery.

When the muscle is very weak, active exercises are given, using buoyancy as an assistance. As power increases, buoyancy is used as a support, and with further recovery, as a form of resistance. This fine progression is invaluable in paralysis of muscle where the muscles retain little power but there is a good range of joint movement, and during recovery, the difficulty of the exercise can be increased very gradually.

A muscle graded as 1 on the Oxford scale (Table 1) can perform movement with buoyancy assisting; as the flicker of movement becomes stronger the exercise can be progressed, using buoyancy as a support; by the time that muscle is graded as 2, it can work against buoyancy. As the power increases to grade 3 and then to grade 4, so the resistance of buoyancy is increased by lengthening the weight-arm of the lever and by adding floats.

Table 1. Scales of muscle power

The Oxford scale of muscle power (on land)	Modification of scale in water
0 = No contraction	1 = Contraction with buoyancy assisting
1 = A flicker of movement	
2 = Movement with gravity counterbalanced	2 = Contraction with buoyancy counterbalanced
3 = Movement against gravity	2+ = Contraction against buoyancy
4 = Movement against gravity and resistance	
5 = Normal	3 = Contraction against buoyancy at speed
	4 = Contraction against buoyancy + light float
	5 = Contraction against buoyancy + heavy float

Note—Grade 5 in water is not normal as normal function cannot be tested there.

Alteration in tone. Tone may be increased, decreased or lost completely. Increased tone is due either to lack of inhibition of anterior horn cell activity, because of an upper motor neurone lesion (e.g. spasticity in hemiplegia), or to irritation of the excitatory part of the reticular formation (e.g. rigidity in Parkinson's Disease).

Spasticity is characterized by an increase in muscle tone in patterns of movement, e.g. flexor spasticity. Another characteristic is that the resistance to passive movement is greatest at the beginning of the range and gradually diminishes.

During pool therapy, the warmth of the water helps to relieve spasticity, even if the relief is only temporary. However, as the spasticity diminishes, passive movements can be given in a greater range and with less discomfort to the patient. In this way joint range can be maintained.

Passive movements should be performed slowly and rhythmically starting with the trunk and proximal joints, gradually including distal joints. The movements should first be of a swinging nature and then of a rotatory nature. The trunk and limbs should be moved in reflex inhibiting movement patterns. The patient should breathe deeply and calmly and the timing of maximum stretch should coincide with expiration. The chief difficulty is to obtain a stable fixation for both patient and therapist. In some instances a second physiotherapist may be needed to assist.

Rigidity is characterized by increased tone in all muscles of the affected part of the body, and resistance is maintained throughout the whole range of passive movement. The warmth of the water and the relaxation it brings reduces rigidity and the limbs are more easily moved, both actively and passively. The movements should, if possible, be actively assisted in movement patterns that 'open' the patient. Again it is important to include trunk movements, especially in the cervical and thoracic spines.

Decreased tone (hypotonia) and flaccidity (loss of tone) results from decreased excitability of the anterior horn cells. Disease or damage affecting the final common pathway leads to flaccidity, as in anterior poliomyelitis and peripheral nerve injuries. As a result of the reduction in tone, voluntary movement is either lost or impaired, and as the affected muscles offer little protection to the joints they are easily damaged.

Formation of contracture and loss of joint movement. Contractures and deformities hamper recovery of voluntary power. They result from the contracture of fibrosed joint structures, or adaptive shortening of the muscles due to muscle imbalance. This is seen in the typical hemiplegic arm or in contracture of the calf muscles following paralysis of the anterior tibial muscles. The resulting stiff joints limit voluntary movement.

When voluntary muscle power is absent, relaxed passive movements are used to prevent contractures and to maintain joint range.

A full range of movement is essential, but if this is limited by pain, the movement should be carried through as great a range as possible. If contractures have developed, controlled stretching is given within the limits of pain, the warmth of the water making the procedure far less painful than on dry land. As soon as voluntary power begins to return, active exercises replace the passive movements.

Loss of coordination. Coordination of movement depends on the correct correlation of all the pathways of the nervous system, and the resulting harmonious working of muscle groups. If any of the pathways are damaged, incoordination develops. Two types of incoordination are sensory and cerebellar ataxia. In sensory ataxia the patient is unaware of the position of his limbs in space unless he uses his vision to see where they are. In cerebellar ataxia the controlling influence of the cerebellum is lost, and hence the inability to perform a smooth, purposeful movement.

Incoordination associated with muscle weakness and spasticity responds to hydrotherapy, but patients with sensory or cerebellar ataxia seem to derive little benefit. While a normal person finds it hard to retain his balance in water—owing partly to buoyancy and partly to the turbulence created by movement—the ataxic patient has even more difficulty, which is intensified by the visual effect of refraction distorting the limbs under water.

Loss of normal postural reflex mechanism and balance. A normal postural reflex mechanism is the basis for normal voluntary and skilled movement. There are three groups of automatic postural reactions:

(*a*) Righting reactions are automatic movements which serve to maintain and restore the normal position of the head in space in its normal relationship to the body, and the normal alignment of trunk and limbs.

(*b*) Equilibrium reactions are automatic movements which serve to maintain and restore balance during all our activities. These postural adjustments to changes of gravity are continuous while we move, and even the smallest changes of equilibrium has to be countered by muscle tone changes. These have to be quick, adequate in range and well timed.

(*c*) Adaptive changes in muscle tone as a protection against the forces of gravity. They can be observed in the trunk and limbs and they overlap to some extent with equilibrium reactions.

There is impairment or loss of the postural reflexes, especially in hemiplegic patients. With the reduction of spasticity in the water and the increase of muscle power, patient's postural reflexes may improve. Overactivity of the sound side has to be curtailed. The patient should be helped to use the affected limbs as early as possible for support and weight bearing. Movements should be initiated from the trunk to activate the affected side or part of the body.

Treatment is started with rhythmic stabilizations being given to the trunk in float lying. Balance exercises—changing the position of the arms and the head—are given in the sitting, and finally in the standing, position. Progression can be made by using turbulence and speed. When head control is impaired or lost, the body can be held in a ball shape (Fig. 11.7) and rocked gently forwards and backwards around the centre of buoyancy. The movements should be equal to the degree of head control, starting with a minute movement away from the vertical in the forward and backward directions. As control improves the swing can be increased.

Circulatory impairment. Loss of voluntary movement leads to loss of pumping action of the muscles, and so the circulation is diminished. This impairs the nutrition of all structures, including the skin and affected muscles.

During hydrotherapy the warmth of the water dilates superficial blood vessels, producing a faint reddening of the skin; this vasodilatation improves the blood supply, and thus helps to prevent impaired nutrition of the skin. Great care must be taken in handling patients with trophic changes; this is particularly important in the water, because the skin breaks down easily and is slow to heal. The deeper circulation can be helped by movement—active when possible, or passive movements of larger joints.

The pressure of the water is directly proportional to its depth. If an oedematous limb is suspended in water, the pressure exerted on the foot is greater than on the thigh. The resulting difference in lateral pressure forces the oedema upwards. The improvement in circulation is clearly evident in the change in colour of the limbs during treatment.

Pain. Pain hampers voluntary movement, and occurs for several reasons. The usual causes are stretching of the contractures during treatment, active inflammation in the nerve sheaths or meninges, and the accumulation of metabolites as a result of impaired circulation due to loss of pumping action of the muscles. Both the warmth and the support of the water help to relieve pain. As the pain is eased care must be taken not to overstretch the contractures during passive movements, as this will intensify the pain.

HEMIPLEGIA

A paralysis of one side of the body, which may also involve the face of the same or opposite side, is known as hemiplegia.

Adult hemiplegia is caused by vascular lesions, such as cerebral haemorrhage, embolism or thrombosis, by tumours, following brain surgery or trauma. The clinical picture shows many variations depending on the degree and distribution of spasticity and on the type of associated sensory disturbance. The features common to most cases of hemiplegia are (a) sensory disturbance of varying degree; (b) spasticity; (c) a disorder of the normal postural reflex mechanism; and (d) loss of selective movement patterns.

Initially the limbs are flaccid, and the patient may be unconscious, but many cases progress to a second stage—the onset of spasticity. It is at this stage that the patient will start pool treatment. This should always be in conjunction with land treatment and should not replace it.

The patient is allowed into the pool when his blood pressure has returned to a reasonable level and when further damage by haemorrhage is no longer likely; generally this would be three to four weeks after the cerebral accident, or even earlier if it is caused by a thrombosis.

The patient is lowered slowly into the pool by the hoist. A momentary rise in blood pressure will occur owing to vasoconstriction as he enters the pool, but this is followed almost immediately by vasodilatation, causing a fall in blood pressure. The physiotherapist must stay with the patient at all times, watching for signs of distress (i.e. breathlessness and sweating on the face).

The first treatment lasts 5 to 10 minutes. For this initial session he is placed in head support lying and then progressed to float support lying, and he is encouraged to relax and become used to the feeling of weightlessness and adjust to body imbalance. Breathing exercises may be given and the patient is instructed to blow out if at any time his face becomes submerged (see Chapter 11).

AIMS OF TREATMENT
1. Reduction of spasticity.
2. Restoration and maintenance of mobility.
3. Inhibition of abnormal patterns of movement and re-education of normal voluntary movement.
4. Improvement of balance and re-education of postural reflexes.
5. Encouragement of swimming and independence.

The techniques used vary according to the distribution of spasticity and the recovery of voluntary movement; therefore a thorough examination is absolutely necessary. Passive movements are given in reflex-inhibiting postures to reduce flexor spasticity in the trunk and arm and extensor or flexor spasticity in the leg. Shakings may be added to the passive movements to enhance the effect of reducing spasticity. The movements are performed with the patient supported on a plinth, and should be carried out slowly and rhythmically. They are given within the limits of pain, as any forced movement will result in increased spasticity.

SUGGESTED PROCEDURES
In ½ sup. ly;
Following shaking, the affected arm is held by the therapist in a reflex-inhibiting position as far as is possible—i.e. shoulder abduction, lateral rotation and extension; elbow extension; forearm supination; wrist extension and abduction; fingers and thumb extension and abduction.

In this position the pelvis and legs are moved passively to the unaffected side and returned to the middle.

Following this, with the patient in the same position, the knees and hips are flexed and the pelvis is rolled passively from side to side.

In ½ sup. s. ly; (on unaffected side)
The therapist places one hand behind the scapula and the other hand on the palm of the patient's hand. From this position she performs rhythmical passive movements of the scapula into protraction and encourages the patient to push his hand forwards.

Ball positioning (Fig. 11.7)
When the patient can hold the arm in protraction, shoulder flexion and elbow wrist and finger extension, he is ready to try the ball position. This means that he moves off the plinth with his knees and

hips flexed and his hands clasped round the anterior aspect of his lower legs. This is particularly valuable for the hemiplegic patient because it is stable for balance and positions the limbs in reflex-inhibiting postures. Once in the ball position, the patient may be rocked forwards and backwards around the centre of buoyancy, starting with small-range movements and gradually increasing the range.

In ½ sup. ly;
The arm is turned out into shoulder lateral rotation with the elbow and hand held in extension and the therapist instructs the patient to carry the arm repeatedly into abduction. The therapist provides assistance as necessary.

In ½ sup. s. ly; (on affected side)
The arm is positioned forward with scapular protraction and elbow extension. The affected leg is in hip extension and the patient is encouraged to bend and stretch the knee—assisted as necessary by the therapist.

In ½ sup. ly;
With the affected arm in an inhibiting position and the knee in flexion, the patient is encouraged to perform flexion and extension of the hip.

Rolling and forward recovery
The patient is encouraged to change from the lying position to the upright position. He bends his head, trunk, hips and knees, brings his arms forward and blows out; this brings the body upright and he can stand. This is progressed by teaching the patient rolling from side to side which encourages trunk rotation, body control and balance. To teach rolling, for example to the right, the patient is in lying and the left foot is crossed over the right foot and the patient rolls over fairly slowly.

The physiotherapist must always face the patient and have him rolling towards her. If the patient requires any assistance he is supported in the lumbar region. For a faster roll, turn by crossing the left arm over the trunk and for an even faster movement, turn by using the head, left arm and left foot.

If the limbs are spastic the physiotherapist should touch the patient as little as possible to prevent the spasticity from being increased.

Sitting (feet on floor and equal weight on buttocks)
The patient pushes down on his hands. This helps to re-educate the action of transfers, because buoyancy is assisting the movement, and it is a good position for the arms due to the fact that it reverses the abnormal pattern.

The patient next moves his arms forwards, sideways, forwards and down. This helps to inhibit the abnormal arm pattern and starts to re-educate sitting balance.

Sitting to standing
The patient can place his hands on the therapist's shoulders but his elbows should stay extended and he must not grip or pull with his hands. The therapist must stand with a wide base and with her shoulders just below water level, bending the knees if necessary to achieve this position.

The patient is then encouraged to stand from sitting, keeping his hips well forward and the affected knee on slight flexion. Once he is standing, turbulence is created by the therapist moving her forearms around his pelvis. This improves standing balance.

When the patient is able to stand, still with the knee in slight flexion and both feet flat on the floor, weight transference from side to side and then backwards and forwards may be practised. Progression is achieved by reducing support from two hands to one hand to standing unsupported. To encourage the patient to take weight through the affected leg, approximation may be applied through the hip or the shoulder with the patient in walk standing (affected foot forwards). The therapist applies a slight backward stretch to the pelvis on the affected side and then encourages the patient to carry his pelvis forwards. This helps to re-educate the stance phase of walking when the patient must have the pelvis vertically above the foot.

Walking
Once he has mastered weight transference, re-education of walking is started. The buoyancy of the water will help to flex the hip and knee and counteract dragging of the leg. The patient should always begin by stepping forwards with the unaffected leg. The support

from the therapist may be as for weight transference. Alternatively, the therapist may walk beside the patient's affected side, supporting in the following manner.

For a left-sided hemiplegia. The therapist's right hand is placed behind the patient's pelvis and her left hand holds the patient's left hand so that his arm is in a reflex-inhibiting position. Her right thigh is placed behind the patient's left hip and knee, to keep his pelvis forward and his knee slightly flexed during the stance phase of walking. As the gait pattern improves, support is reduced.

Weight transference and walking will prove to be difficult in the water if the leg is very flaccid as the therapist cannot facilitate proprioception through the heel and knee because of buoyancy and turbulence.

Balance can be improved by the patient maintaining a position while the physiotherapist creates turbulence around him. The position will progress from lying to sitting and to standing, and as his balance improves it will help with walking and swimming.

Swimming and games
Swimming plays a great part in the re-education of coordination. Prowess at swimming depends greatly on the amount of voluntary power and the patient's ability to swim prior to the disability. Swimming is taught following the Halliwick principles (see Chapters 11 and 7).

When the hemiplegic patient lies on his back there is a tendency to roll to the affected side because of the body asymmetry. This can be counteracted by the patient turning his head to the unaffected side. When the patient can balance in the floating position, he is then encouraged to begin swimming.

At first, he will tend to swim in circles because of the unequal pull of the unaffected arm and leg. When lying on his back this will result in a left-sided hemiplegic turning in a circle to the left. To swim in a straight line the affected right hand is placed behind the back, thereby causing turbulence which will keep the body moving straight backwards. As he improves, this tendency becomes less apparent, and the patient finds encouragement in his ability to perform some recreational activity. The type of swimming stroke will depend on the patient's previous swimming ability. It is easier to start on the back using bilateral back stroke with the arms two-thirds elevated. If the arms are fully elevated the body tends to sink and will eventually roll until it is face downwards.

Games in which various sizes of ball are pushed through the water are used to re-educate balance, and are given in sitting or standing positions, depending on the ability of the patient to balance. Competition games should be avoided as they increase the use of effort and, with it, increase spasticity.

Pool treatment should always be in conjunction with land treatment and should not replace it.

PARAPLEGIA AND TETRAPLEGIA

Paralysis of both lower limbs may follow trauma such as dislocation at certain levels of the thoracic or lumbar vertebrae, possibly with associated fractures; or may be due to disease such as tumour, bone disease or transverse myelitis causing damage to the spinal cord or the cauda equina. If the lesion is above the level of the first thoracic vertebra the arms will be involved also, causing a tetraplegia. A lesion at any higher level, as in the upper thoracic region, will cause respiratory impairment due to paralysis of intercostal and abdominal muscles, and any lesion above the fifth cervical vertebra will result in diaphragmatic involvement and severe respiratory distress.

Patients with a vital capacity as low as 1 litre should be treated with care, and if signs of respiratory distress develop they should probably not be treated in the pool.

There will also be vasomotor disturbances due to the involvement of the autonomic nervous system, causing loss of vasoconstriction. This means that the patient is liable to faint in the pool, especially on sitting up from the lying position. If the lesion is below the first lumbar vertebra the cauda equina is involved, and the lesion is of the lower motor neurone type; if above, an upper motor neurone lesion will result.

Recovery will depend on the extent of the damage: with complete severance of the cord no voluntary power will return, but if the severance is incomplete or if symptoms are due to pressure some return of voluntary power can be expected.

Following trauma a patient will be given hydrotherapy when the fracture or dislocation has consolidated, which will be in about eight to twelve weeks. The stage at which hydrotherapy is indicated for paraplegia due to disease must be dictated by the nature of the disease.

The patient may suffer from some degree of incontinence, so his bladder must be emptied before entering the pool, and it must be ascertained that his bowels have been emptied that day. Some patients may be catheterized, in which case the catheter is spigotted and pool treatment can be given. To prevent any contamination of the water, the level of chlorination can be stepped up or treatment given at the end of the day.

At first the patient is lowered into the pool by hoist. As sufficient voluntary movement recovers and muscle power improves he can be taught to use a pulley, and swing himself into the pool. Later still he can be transferred from his wheelchair to the edge of the pool and he will enter it from there. The physiotherapist must, however, always be at hand to give help and to prevent accidents.

AIMS OF TREATMENT

1. Reduction of spasticity and prevention of contractures.
2. Improvement of vital capacity and breathing control.
3. Hypertrophy of the unaffected muscle groups.
4. Improvement of the patient's balance.
5. Teaching swimming and recreational activities, thereby improving morale.

TREATMENT

The treatment starts with the patient in float lying and the therapist provides manual fixation behind the scapulae. The therapist then applies pressure to the patient's trunk so that his legs swing from side to side as she walks backwards. The slow rhythmical swinging movements help to relax the patient and reduce spasticity.

Passive movements. Passive movements are performed with the patient in $\frac{1}{2}$ sup. ly. and fixed securely by a strap or a second therapist. The movements should be slow and rhythmical, starting with trunk rotation and side flexion; proceeding to lower-limb movements from hip to knee to foot. Trunk passive movements with breathing as described in Chapter 7 are useful for these patients.

Two joint muscles such as gastrocnemius or rectus femoris should be stretched slowly, held for a few seconds, then slowly released. This is to prevent contractures.

Active movements. Active exercises are given for the muscles which retain normal innervation, i.e. arm and trunk muscles in paraplegic patients. Particular attention is paid to strengthening the shoulder extensors and adductors and the elbow extensors, as these are the arm muscles needed for crutch walking. Resistance is used in the form of bats and floats. Trunk exercises to strengthen all innervated muscle groups are given and are progressed by adding floats and rings. Fixation of the trunk, by using the arms, helps in strengthening both arm and trunk muscles.

EXERCISES
The following are examples of exercises which may be given.
1. gr. fl. sup. ly; (bats)—A press d. (shoulder extensors).
2. yd. gr. fl. sup. ly; (bats)—A press d. (shoulder retractors).
3. gr. ½ sup. pr. ly; T push away with Elb. straighten and pull f. with Elb. bend. Manual resistance may be given at thighs (Fig. 9.1).
4. gr. fl. sup. ly; (bats)—A raise s. and lower. As the arms are moved the physiotherapist resists first forward and then backward movement of the body at the feet.

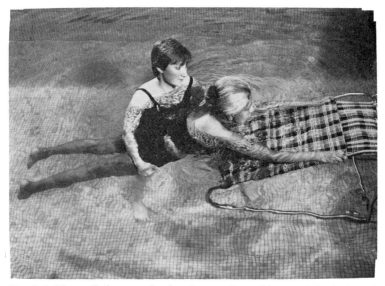

Fig. 9.1. Upper limb strengthening for a patient with a partial spinal cord compression lesion.

5. gr. sitt; (floats)—A push d. and relax.
6. ½ sup. ly; L swing s. to s. (trunk side flexors and latissimus dorsi).
7. hve. gr. ly; T swing s. to s.
8. ½ sup. ly; L push d. (trunk extensors).
9. rch. gr. sitt; (bats)—T turn s. to s. (trunk rotators esp. oblique abdo. mm).
10. sitt; breast stroke arm movts.
11. fl. sup. ly; Pelvis push d. into water (trunk flexors).
12. Stabilizations to the trunk in float lying.

PATTERNS OF MOVEMENT
All arm patterns are useful (see Chapter 7). The trunk side-flexion and flexion–extension patterns are also beneficial.

For tetraplegic patients some of the exercises are not possible, e.g. exercises 8, 9, 11 and 12.

Balance. This will depend on the site of the lesion, and is less affected if the abdominal muscles are not involved, as with lesions occurring below the thoracic vertebrae. Vision plays a great part in maintaining balance, as the patient has no idea of the position in space of his body under water. With the patient in float support lying, the physiotherapist moves the trunk from side to side while the patient tries to remain steady. The range of movement is decreased gradually until all muscle groups are working at once, giving a stabilizing effect.

Balance is taught in sitting with the patient holding on to the seat. He then lifts one arm forwards, then sideways. As his balance improves both arms are lifted forwards and then sideways. Turbulence of the water is used as a further progression. As balance can be upset by turbulence the physiotherapist must be careful not to walk too quickly round the patient as this may cause him to overbalance.

Standing
When the patient can sit unaided he can begin to learn to stand. He is taught to stand and lock his knee joints by extending the hips (Fig. 9.2). If he cannot do this, a polythene back splint can be bandaged to the knees for support.

Standing is taught first in the parallel bars, the patient holding on to the therapist or to the rail of the pool. The physiotherapist stands

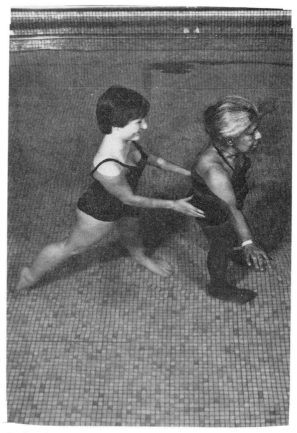

Fig. 9.2. Patient learning to balance in standing. Same patient as in Fig. 9.1.

facing the patient and supports the pelvis, while the patient rests his hands on her shoulders or forearms. The degree of proficiency in walking again depends on the level of the lesion; with lower lesions the use of the abdominal muscles is retained, but this is not so with the higher level lesions when only the latissimus dorsi muscles are working. If the patient has the use of his abdominal muscles, a swing-to gait, and later a swing-through gait, are taught. When the abdominal muscles are paralysed the patient is taught to hitch his legs forward, using the lattissimus dorsi muscles. Owing to buoyancy, lifting the body up is easier than on land, but the legs tend to float away. The physiotherapist can control the pelvis by assisting or resisting the movements where necessary and this will improve the patient's walking.

Swimming and games
Swimming is taught from the beginning, initially from a remedial aspect but later as a recreational activity (Fig. 9.3). It helps to improve the patient's strength, mobility, coordination and respiratory control, in addition to boosting his morale. The legs have a tendency to float but the feet are lower in the water than the rest of the body. To counteract this the paraplegic patient has to hyperextend his back by using his arm and trunk muscles in order to keep his head above the water.

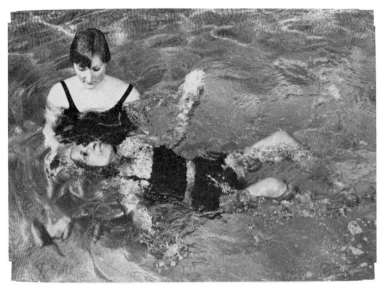

Fig. 9.3. Swimming on back. Same patient as Figs 9.1. and 9.2.

Floating on the back is the easiest position for the patient and he is taught to control his body from sitting upright to floating and back again. Sculling with arms is taught first; then the arms are lifted slowly up and out of the water and then down quickly through the water, thus providing the propelling force. Progression is made from double-arm back crawl to alternate arm back crawl. The difficulty with the latter is that with every stroke of the arm the trunk and pelvis rotate because the paralysed legs cannot counteract the movement. This can be prevented by a sculling action with the arm that is in the water.

The patient learns rolling from supine to prone by turning the head to one side and following it with the opposite arm. The patient must be taught to blow out when the face is submerged. Swimming in the prone position is more difficult, especially front crawl. Patients with lower lesions will be able to swim in this position but those with cervical lesions will have difficulty. Patients with low cervical lesions can become proficient in the breast stroke but only a few can manage the front crawl. These patients are taught to swim a few strokes with the head down in the water and then to hyperextend the neck to bring the head out of the water whenever they need to breathe.

Games like water polo bring a lot of fun and at the same time improve control and speed of reaction.

MULTIPLE SCLEROSIS

This is a chronic disease of unknown aetiology affecting the white matter of the brain cerebellum and spinal cord. The signs and symptoms depend on the site of the lesion, but can be divided into three basic groups—upper motor neurone, cerebellar and sensory. The groups are not clearly defined, however, as most patients show mixed signs with one group predominating. Patients in the cerebellar and sensory groups gain less benefit from pool therapy than do those in whom upper motor neurone symptoms of spasticity predominate. The nerve fibres passing to the lower limbs have a longer course, so that the most commonly treated form is that of spasticity affecting both lower limbs.

As many of the patients, particularly the advanced cases, suffer from incontinence, care must be taken to see that the bladder is emptied before entering the pool or the catheter is spigotted off. Provided there is no infection, incontinence does not present too much difficulty.

The aims of treatment are similar to those for the hemiplegic patient, and include reduction of spasticity, prevention of contractures and re-education of voluntary power and functional activities, including walking. In advanced cases, the pool is of great value in relieving the pain arising from spasticity, and since this may be the only place where the patient is relatively free from pain, the physiotherapist may well find she has an eager and cooperative patient.

For descriptive purposes treatment is divided into early and advanced stages.

EARLY STAGE

Relaxed passive movements in patterns are given to prevent contractures from developing. Exercises for the legs are introduced to improve coordination and to break up the abnormal pattern. As the condition is progressive, the patient may become chair-bound, so the emphasis is to strengthen the arms, making him as independent as possible.

With the lower limbs in reflex-inhibiting positions, arm and trunk exercises are given, with particular emphasis on the latissimus dorsi, elbow extensors and all the trunk muscles. Functional activities such as walking, climbing stairs, sitting down and standing up, transferring from one surface to another and stepping on and off a small step can all be given in water. The relief of weight by buoyancy makes it possible for these patients to walk in the water when muscle weakness and spasticity makes this impossible on land. The morale of the patient can be raised by recreational activities such as swimming, but care must be taken not to overtire the patient.

ADVANCED STAGE

By this stage the patient may be in considerable pain from contractures that have developed owing to spasticity and muscle imbalance. Relaxation is encouraged with the patient completely supported in the water by floats. The warmth of the water and the support aids this relaxation, and passive movements and stretching of contractures can then be given. In some instances a second physiotherapist is required to steady the patient. Any remaining voluntary movement should be encouraged, but care should be taken not to overtire him. By now the patient will probably be completely chairbound and unable to walk, even in the pool. The relief of pain and the freedom of movement provided by the pool is of great psychological value apart from the beneficial effects of the treatment.

SUGGESTED EXERCISES

The following are suggested exercises for a patient with predominantly upper motor neurone signs affecting both legs. These are a guide to the type of exercises that might be given, selection depending on requirements of individual patients.

1. fl. sup. ly; general relaxation.
2. fl. sup. ly; relaxed passive movements to lower limbs in pattern; e.g.
   (a) 1 Hip and K flexion with plantar flexion, 1 Hip and K extension with dorsiflexion.
   (b) L abduct. with medial rotation and adduct. with lateral rotation.
3. ½ sup. ly; (patient grasps sides of plinth)—L swing s. to s.
4. ½ sup. s. ly; Hip and K bend and relax.
5. ½ gr. st; alt. Hip and K bend and stretch.
6. sitt; change to st. then back to sitt.
7. bd. sitt; Elb. straighten and bend. Progress by adding floats in the hand.
8. sitt; transfer along form or to other seat.
9. ½ sup. pr. ly; K bend up under stretcher and relax.
10. st; walk forw. and sidew.
11. fl. sup. ly; A raise s. to yd. and b. Progress by adding bats.
12. fl. sup. ly; A push d. into water and b. Progress by adding bats.
13. ly; teach balance. Balancing must be taught as for hemiplegia.
14. ly; teach rolling.

When scissoring occurs, lateral rotation or rolling should be taught first.

Encourage swimming on the back at first and progress to swimming on the face.

PARKINSONISM

Parkinsonism is a syndrome characterized by muscular rigidity and tremor resulting in poor voluntary movement and impaired posture and balance. These clinical features are also evident in the degenerative condition known as Parkinson's disease. Treatment in the pool can be very helpful in 'loosening' the patient. Rigidity will be reduced owing to the physiological effects of the warm water, thereby facilitating movement.

AIMS OF TREATMENT
1. Reduction of rigidity.
2. Improvement or maintenance of joint mobility.
3. Improvement of posture by encouraging extension movements.
4. Increase of thoracic expansion.
5. Re-education of gait.

Some patients with Parkinson's disease prefer a cold to a hot environment; in these cases land treatment would be more suitable.

TECHNIQUES
The patient starts in ½ sup. crk. ly; and the therapist rolls his knees passively from side to side to gain relaxation. The movements must be performed rhythmically, and as relaxation occurs the sweep is increased until full range is obtained.

When nearly full range has been obtained the patient is encouraged to join in the movement actively.

Then with the patient sitting, trunk rotation is again performed. The patient's arms are held with the hands clasped, elbows extended and shoulders in 90° flexion. The therapist assists the patient to move his arms from side to side, increasing the range of trunk rotation and again with the patient joining in as much as possible, provided that the movement is smooth and rhythmical.

With the patient in float lying and the therapist fixing the pelvis, trunk side-flexion may be performed passively, slowly and rhythmically, with a gradual increase in range and the patient joining in actively. The lower trunk may be moved if the patient is in neck-rest fl. ly; and the therapist fixes the elbows. The patient's legs then swing from side to side. As the range is increased, trunk rotation may be incorporated with the patient instructed to lead with his heels. If the patient cannot place his arms in the neck-rest position, the therapist fixes on the scapulae.

Trunk flexion and extension with rotation (Chapter 7) may also be used. Trunk movements with breathing exercises are also indicated (Chapter 7). All of the foregoing activities should be performed equally to both sides and counting may help to maintain a smooth rhythm.

Trunk rotation may also be practised with the patient in $\frac{1}{2}$ sup. std. ly. He is instructed to carry one leg over the other, alternating to each side, with the therapist assisting.

Walking is easier in the water than on land. The therapist may need to help with initiation of movement, but the resistance of the water impedes the festinating gait which so many patients have on land. If the therapist walks in front of the patient fairly quickly, her wake helps to initiate the patient's walking.

Many patients enjoy swimming which improves coordination and balance and they should be taught to roll and blow out in the water when the face is submerged. Lateral rotation of the body is achieved by the patient's bringing one arm or leg across the trunk, turning the head in the direction of the roll, when the body will automatically turn. If the patient cannot carry the arm across the trunk, then if he lifts the arm out of the water he will roll to the side of that arm.

POLYNEUROPATHY

This condition affects the nerve fibres of the brain stem and many peripheral nerves. There is degeneration of the myelin sheath and axons of the cranial and spinal nerves resulting in widespread muscle weakness and wasting with alteration or loss of sensation.

The disease is usually bilateral and symmetrical with the initial symptoms in the hands and feet, because the distal parts of the nerves are affected first. The tendon reflexes in the affected limbs are absent. In some cases the paralysis can extend beyond the limbs involving the trunk muscles and including the respiratory, neck and face muscles.

The majority of patients with polyneuritis recover if either the cause has been found and eliminated early in the toxic type, or if they have survived the respiratory paralysis following the acute infective type. In this type the onset is sudden, beginning with a febrile illness followed by a paralytic stage. The paralysis is of the lower motor neurone type with flaccid muscles. In many cases the paralysis spreads for two to three weeks, then remains stationary for a few weeks and then begins to recover. After the acute phase there is symmetrical paralysis of certain muscle groups.

In the acute and active stages of the disease, and especially if there is evidence of myocarditis, bed rest is essential. The patient is allowed into the pool when the first signs of recovery become apparent. Patients with respiratory involvement are allowed in the pool, provided they do not suffer from respiratory distress. As there is a long period of recovery the patient needs encouragement and reassurance. This recovery period must be expected to last for at least 6 months and may well continue for a year.

The affected muscles are tested out of water and are charted on the Oxford scale, and also in water using the modified scale (page 126).

AIMS OF TREATMENT
1. Improvement of circulation and reduction of swelling.
2. Prevention of contractures and deformities.
3. Re-education of the affected muscles and maintenance of strength of the unaffected muscles.
4. Improvement of thoracic expansion.
5. Re-education of balance.
6. Restoration to as full function as possible.

Owing to the paralysis, circulation is poor and the skin is oedematous and sweating. The warm water improves the circulation and so the nutrition to the skin and muscles, helps to reduce swelling, and warms the muscles so enabling them to work more effectively. It is important that the affected muscles should not be stretched, but full-range movements must be maintained in all joints. If the muscles are too weak to produce active movements, then relaxed passive movements are carried out to prevent contractures, and to maintain joint range and circulation.

TREATMENT
The scheme of treatment will vary from patient to patient. Strengthening exercises are given to the unaffected muscles using buoyancy as a resistance or with the manually resisted movement patterns described in Chapter 7. The proximal muscles of the limbs and those of the trunk are worked hard to get overflow into the affected muscles.

EXERCISES

Examples are the following:

1. H sup. ly; L push d. into water with B arch. This works the back extensors against buoyancy and encourages extension in the hips, knees and plantar flexor muscles. Progress by adding float to lower legs.
2. fl. sup. s. ly; flex. and ext. trunk patterns (Chapter 7).
3. fl. sup. ly; trunk side-flex. patterns (Chapter 7).
4. breathing exercises with trunk movements as in Chapter 7.

A carefully graded progression is used for all affected muscles, the starting point and the rate of progression depending on the individual patient. The fine progression of resistance provided by buoyancy gives an ideal method for strengthening weakened muscles, but great care must be taken in the early stages not to tire them. Trick movements like hitching of the hip during leg abduction must be avoided, at least until there is no further hope of recovery.

If the quadriceps are weak the following are examples of the progressive exercises that may be given.

1. $\frac{1}{2}$ sup. ly; (float round K)—1K straighten. Here buoyancy is assisting but the range is small.
2. sitt; 1K straighten. Here buoyancy is assisting but the range is greater. The physiotherapist returns the leg to the starting position.
3. $\frac{1}{2}$ sup. s. ly; 1K straighten and bend. Buoyancy is counterbalanced. Progress by increasing the range, speed, repetitions or adding a flipper.
4. $\frac{1}{2}$ st; (with K bent back)—1K straighten and bend (buoyancy resisting).

If the patient is unable to stand, then the exercises in $\frac{1}{2}$ sup. s. ly; can be further progressed by adding unstreamlined floats. Progression in standing is made by adding floats, increasing the speed and repetitions.

5. $\frac{1}{2}$ st; 1 Hip and 1K extension push d. float into water. This is a functional exercise working both hip and knee extensor muscles strongly against buoyancy.

Walking, swimming and games

Walking in the pool is hampered at first because the patient has difficulty in controlling the legs against buoyancy. When he can manage to keep his feet on the floor, gait training may begin as in Chapter 7.

Recreational activities play a big part in maintaining the patient's morale, as well as strengthening his muscles generally and keeping him mobile. All the swimming strokes provide valuable exercise, from the simplest sculling movements to the more advanced breast stroke and crawl. Competitive games such as swimming are encouraged provided the patients are at more or less the same stage of recovery. Once the patient can swim safely by himself, he should be encouraged to go to the local baths or to join a swimming club, though he must be warned of the difference in the temperature of the water. Unless he can keep moving the colder water will cause discomfort and may therefore discourage him from further effort.

At first the patient can do more in the pool than on land and this is of psychological value. Later, when he can do more on land he is encouraged to work still harder to achieve even better results.

PERIPHERAL NERVE LESIONS

Damage to a peripheral nerve results in a lower motor neurone lesion. The chief effects of these lesions are loss of muscle power, muscle atrophy, stiff joints and deformity, impaired circulation, and trophic changes. Treatment in the pool is useful in maintaining the circulation, thereby reducing the trophic changes, in maintaining joint mobility and in facilitating the re-education of returning muscle power.

The extent of the signs and symptoms will depend on the site and severity of the lesion.

When surgical repair is necessary a patient will not be allowed in the pool until the sutures have been removed and the wound is fully healed. With all lesions care must be taken not to damage the skin and the area of the lesion must be dried carefully after every treatment.

Passive movements are given to all the affected joints to prevent deformity, and, together with the warmth of the water, will maintain the circulation. The warmth of the water also makes the movement more comfortable. Unaffected muscle groups are worked strongly in suitable arm or leg patterns to facilitate the contraction of the paralysed muscles. For example, in a lesion of the common peroneal nerve, hip and knee flexors can be used to facilitate the dorsi-flexor muscles of the ankle. Once a contraction is initiated active exercises can be given to the muscles using buoyancy as an assistance, as a support and finally as a resistance. The affected muscles can be treated using the grading as described in the treatment of polyneuropathy.

Exercises for specific muscles may be better given on land where fixation assists in localization of movement.

When the lesion affects only a hand or a foot the limb can be immersed in a warm bath instead of the patient being treated in the pool. Where the lesion is caused by a fracture or dislocation, pool therapy has a greater part to play in the patient's rehabilitation.

BRACHIAL PLEXUS LESIONS

A lesion of the brachial plexus may be complete or partial, lesions of the upper trunk being most common. In complete lesions sensation is lost entirely and all muscles in the upper limb except the trapezius muscle are paralysed, causing the limb to hang limply with the shoulder medially rotated, the elbow extended and the forearm pronated. The joints are unprotected due to lack of muscle tone and the shoulder may subluxate with little or no force. A combination of gravity and lack of movement will cause the hand to become blue and swollen. Partial lesions of the upper trunk affect the muscles of the shoulder and the elbow flexors, while lesions of the lower trunk affect the muscles of the hand. If the lesion is complete the limb may have to be amputated, but in partial lesions a combination of surgery, splinting and physiotherapy may help to restore function.

Pool therapy is often used in the treatment of partial lesions and begins as soon as the initial shock has worn off and any associated injuries such as fractures or wounds have healed. With the patient in float support lying, passive movements are given to all affected joints, those that counteract the deformity being most important (lateral rotation and abduction of the shoulder, supination of the forearm, flexion of the metacarpophalangeal joints and abduction of the fingers and thumb). Care must be taken to ensure that the shoulder is covered by the water. The patient should sit on a bench of suitable height or be instructed to bend his knees so that his shoulder is fully submerged. By using the fine progression possible with buoyancy, voluntary power can be re-educated. Functional activities involving the use of the whole arm must be encouraged. The following is an outline of progressive treatment for a patient with a partial brachial plexus lesion affecting the upper trunk.

Buoyancy-assisted and neutralized exercises for the shoulder girdle and shoulder muscles
1. fl. sup. ly; relaxed passive movements are described above.
2. sitt; Sh. shrugg. and push d. This is followed by posture correction with emphasis on the level of the shoulder girdle.
3. sitt; A raise s. (returned to starting position by physiotherapist). A common fault with all shoulder injuries is reversed humero-scapular rhythm. Correct rhythm can be established with this exercise.
4. sitt; 1A lift b. (returned to starting position by physiotherapist).
5. fl. sup. ly; A raise s. and lower. If the deltoid muscle is completely paralysed, full abduction and elevation can be performed by rotating the humerus laterally, using biceps and triceps for abduction followed by pectoralis major and serratus anterior to complete the movement.
6. Hnds. clsp. rch. sitt; T turn with A push from s. to s.
7. sitt; (A abd. to rt. angle and Elb. flexed)—1A push f. acr. T and pull b.
8. fwd. lean sitt; 1A raise f. and u. (returned to starting position by therapist).

Exercises 3 and 8 can be progressed by the number of repetitions, by increasing the speed and, as muscle power improves, by strapping floats or bats to the arm.

Later exercises as recovery is taking place
1. ½ yd. sitt; 1 Elb. bend and stretch.
2. sitt; A movements of breast stroke.
3. ½ yd. sitt; 1A push float across water. Float at hand. Progress to pushing small bat.
4. ½ fra. sup. incl. tow. s. st; 1A swing f. and b.
5. ½ gr. incl. tow. s. st; (arm at water level)—1A swing f. and b. Gradually decrease the inclination to increase abduction.

6. rch. sitt; A push d. and b.
7. ½ gr. ½ sup. pr. ly; 1A push d. into water.
8. str. gr. fl. sup. pr. ly; A bend and stretch.
9. Toe sup. ly; A back crawl pattern.
10. fl. sup. ly; sculling.
11. Bad Ragaz A patterns (see Chapter 7).
12. gr. ½ sup. pr. ly; crawl leg action.
13. hve. gr. sup. ly; 1L push d. and relax.

In exercises 12 and 13 the arm muscles are being used to stabilize the trunk.

14. Swimming breast stroke, progress to crawl.

As power in the hand returns, exercises may be progressed by holding bats or floats.

This scheme of treatment is intended only as a guide. The progression will vary with each patient and will be accompanied by treatment in the gymnasium. The final stages of rehabilitation will be carried out in the gymnasium.

10
Treatment of Orthopaedic Conditions

Hydrotherapy is of great value in the rehabilitation of patients with orthopaedic conditions.

The buoyancy of the water allows a fine grading of progression in the strengthening of weak muscles; it helps to increase the range of movement in the larger joints and gives weight relief in the re-education of walking. Owing to the warmth of the water, pain from trauma or following surgery is relieved. Hydrotherapy should always be given in conjunction with, and supplementary to, exercise on dry land.

Balance is assisted by the hydrostatic pressure working on all surfaces of the body.

CLINICAL SIGNS AND SYMPTOMS

Orthopaedic conditions suitable for pool therapy may be characterized by pain, bruising, muscle spasm, swelling, limitation of joint movement, muscle weakness, incoordination, poor balance and abnormal gait.

Pain and muscle spasm. The part that is painful or in muscle spasm is completely immersed in the water and therefore all aspects are warmed. This affect is maintained throughout the treatment. Great care is necessary when the patient is being moved or when floats are being applied in case buoyancy produces a sudden unwanted movement causing pain. Movement of the patient as a whole, however, is very much easier in the pool than on land.

Bruising and swelling. The warmth of the water increases the circulation and therefore helps to disperse the bruising. Swelling may be acute or chronic and can be decreased by the improvement in the circulation and also by the pressure of the water on the limb. This is greater at the bottom of the pool in accordance with Pascal's law. *Limitation of joint movement.* Treatment in the pool is mainly beneficial for stiffness of the larger joints such as the hip, knee, shoulder and the joints of the spine. The range of movement is assessed in the buoyancy supported position. In the early stages of treatment exercises are performed with buoyancy assisting the moving part and in the greatest possible range within the limits of pain. 'Hold–relax' techniques may be used with buoyancy assisting movement into the new range. Oscillatory passive movements (mobilizations) may be used to gain range during the relief of pain and muscle spasm obtained from the warmth and buoyancy of the water. Fixation for some of these techniques may be more difficult than on land but can be provided successfully, manually by a second therapist or by straps.

Muscle weakness. The warmth of the water increases the circulation to the muscles and so improves their function. The re-education of weak muscles can be finely graded from buoyancy-assisted, through buoyancy-counterbalanced to buoyancy-resisted exercises. The muscles can be made to work more strongly by using, for example, turbulence, flippers or floats, but the final rehabilitation may be better carried out on land.

Incoordination and poor balance. Owing to the weight-relieving effect of buoyancy a patient can stand in the pool without support, such as crutches or sticks, before doing so on land. This means that the balance and coordination of the lower limb muscles can be retrained at an earlier stage than on land. Coordination and balance re-education may start in any position according to the requirements of the individual. As the patient's balance improves turbulence can be created, at first by the physiotherapist and then by the patient himself moving his arms. Coordination of the trunk muscles can be improved by giving stabilizations in float support lying. Owing to refraction by the water the part of the body below the water level appears distorted, and therefore posture re-education is difficult in the pool and should be carried out on land. Nevertheless, whenever the patient is in any upright position he must be encouraged to feel that his weight is evenly distributed.

Abnormal gait. Re-education of walking may be started early in the pool. Partial weight-bearing walking is carried out at first in deep water (the water level at the patient's axilla), and as the patient improves the water level is reduced gradually until he is walking in the shallowest part of the pool. There is thus a gradual transition from partial weight-bearing to full weight-bearing. Where a patient has shortening of a lower limb a weighted built-up shoe can be given to him to use in the pool

CONDITIONS RESPONDING TO TREATMENT

Conditions that respond well to pool therapy include:

1. Fractures and dislocations
2. Surgery to large joints and the spine
3. Soft-tissue injuries

In the following outlines the times suggested for pool treatment both initially and within a specific scheme are only approximate indications.

Rehabilitation in the pool after surgery may begin as soon as the sutures are out, usually in 10–14 days. Op-Site is used if the wound is not completely healed.

FRACTURED NECK OF FEMUR

This fracture frequently occurs in the elderly. Whether the fracture is impacted or displaced it is usually treated by surgery. This may be by the insertion of a pin, by a pin and plate or by the total replacement of the head of the femur with a prosthesis. Special care should be taken with an elderly patient and the physiotherapist must reassure the patient and explain carefully the treatment to be given and the reasons for it. The majority of patients will enter the pool by the hoist for the first few treatments, especially if there are a number of steps into the pool.

The aims of treatment are to strengthen the muscles round the hip joint and the quadriceps, to mobilize or maintain mobility in the affected hip and knee, to re-educate walking and to rehabilitate to independence.

The patient performs buoyancy-assisted exercises for the hip abductors lying on his side; for the hip extensor muscles in the prone position; and for the hip flexor muscles or knee extensors in lying. The half stretcher used to support the patient should be sloping. Alternatively, the patient may perform the same movements in inclined side standing, inclined prone standing or inclined standing. For hip flexion or knee extension the patient may be sitting. During all these exercises it is important that the patient's pelvis is stabilized to prevent lumbar spine movements. 'Hold–relax' can be given to any tight group of muscles with buoyancy assisting into the new range. The exercises may then be progressed to the buoyancy-neutralized positions. As the condition of the patient improves exercises can be performed against the resistance of buoyancy. The patient is taught to change from the sitting to the standing position, this being easier than getting up from a chair as buoyancy assists the movement. Walking re-education is included in the programme of treatment from the beginning. Emphasis is put on small even steps correcting any abnormal pattern.

If the patient is elderly swimming will not always be included in the treatment, but the back stroke leg movement can be taught in float support lying. This encourages all movements of the hip. These patients are treated until independence has been achieved with a walking frame or crutches on land, at which time pool treatment may be discontinued.

The following exercises provide a guide to the treatment that may be given after a fractured neck of femur.

INITIAL EXERCISES

1. $\frac{1}{2}$ gr. incl. tow. s. st; 1L raise s. and relax (therapist takes leg back to starting position).
2. gr. incl. pr. st; 1L raise b. and relax (therapist takes leg back to starting position).
3. hve. gr. incl. st; 1L raise f. and relax (therapist returns leg to starting position if necessary).
4. sitt; 1K stretch and bend.
5. $\frac{1}{2}$ sup. s. ly; 1L raise and relax (therapist takes leg back to starting position).
6. $\frac{1}{2}$ sup. pr. ly; 1L raise and relax (therapist takes leg back to starting position).
7. $\frac{1}{2}$ sup. ly; 1K bend and stretch.
   'Hold–relax' can be given to increase abduction and extension of the hip.

8. $\frac{1}{2}$ sup. s. ly; 1K bend and stretch.
9. $\frac{1}{2}$ sup. ly; L part and close.
10. $\frac{1}{2}$ sup. ly; alt. L push d. and relax.
11. $\frac{1}{2}$ sup. K bd. ly; F part (K remain together).

LATER EXERCISES
1. $\frac{1}{2}$ sup. ly; 1L push d. (float at K).
2. rch. gr. st; Hip and K bend and stretch.
3. $\frac{1}{2}$ sup. s. ly; Under L push d. and relax.
4. $\frac{1}{2}$ gr. $\frac{1}{2}$ st; (at rail) 1K bend and straighten.
5. $\frac{1}{2}$ sup. ly; back stroke leg movements.

RESISTED EXERCISES

Where a patient's hip has had a replacement arthroplasty, no strong resisted rotation or abduction beyond midline should be attempted. Free exercises against buoyancy are suitable but floats or flippers should not be added.

Manual resistance may be applied to all muscle groups working isometrically in the neutral position.

Where the surgical management has been by insertion of a pin and plate the patient can be progressed to resisted movements in all directions and in full range.

SUITABLE PATTERNS

All isometric leg patterns are suitable. For patients with a pin and plate, bilateral abduction and adduction patterns and single-leg flex extension patterns may be used.

FRACTURED SHAFT OF FEMUR

These fractures may be treated conservatively by traction or surgically by internal fixation using an intramedullary nail. Pool therapy is of value after both methods and is particularly beneficial if the condition is bilateral as walking can be given at an earlier time than on land. These patients are usually young and the later treatment can be vigorous.

Following surgery pool therapy can begin two to three weeks after the operation. The patient enters the pool by the hoist and only non-weight-bearing exercises are given. The chief aims of treatment are to improve knee and hip mobility, and to strengthen the quadriceps muscle.

INITIAL EXERCISES
1. $\frac{1}{2}$ sup. s. ly; 1K bend and stretch.
2. $\frac{1}{2}$ sup. s. ly; repeated contractions to knee flexors and extensors.
3. $\frac{1}{2}$ sup. s. ly; bicycling action.
4. $\frac{1}{2}$ sup. ly; 1L press d.
5. sitt; 1K straighten and bend.
6. $\frac{1}{2}$ sup. ly; alt. L carry s.
7. $\frac{1}{2}$ sup. ly; L part and clos.
8. $\frac{1}{2}$ sup. ly; alt. L push d.
9. $\frac{1}{2}$ sup. ly; (K bd.) F push apart (K tog.).
10. $\frac{1}{2}$ sup. ly; (K bd.) K push apart (F tog.).

PATTERNS OF MOVEMENT
Trunk side-flexion and isometric hip abduction are suitable patterns to start with.

When these patients are floating the affected limb tends to sink owing to diminished muscle bulk. This makes swimming difficult but back stroke is possible. Breast stroke will be difficult owing to limited hip and knee mobility, but this stroke may be used as a progression on back stroke.

Provided the water is deep enough walking may begin after four weeks. The patient tends to swing the leg from the hip rather than bend the hip and knee and this must be corrected. Walking in the pool is partially weight-bearing and the amount of weight taken by the limb is the weight of that part of the body out of the water. Ideally walking should be progressed by moving from deeper to shallower water. Re-education of walking is carried out as described in Chapter 7. The exercises are progressed by using floats and flippers as resistance and the amount of support in walking is reduced gradually until the patient is allowed to do full weight-bearing on land. This will be any time after 12 weeks, depending on the amount of callus formation.

For later stages of rehabilitation, bilateral hip abduction, extension, abduction and medial rotation of the hip with knee extension, flexion, adduction, lateral rotation of the hip with knee flexion, single-leg abduction, all performed isotonically, are suitable.

With conservative treatment the patient will be on traction for approximately 12 weeks. Knee movements will be very limited and the quadriceps muscles weak after the long period of traction. The patient may begin pool treatment when the period of traction is over but progresses from non-weight-bearing to partial-weight-bearing exercises is one to two weeks. Full weight-bearing is achieved in 4–6 months from the time of injury, again depending on the callus formation.

Swimming. Breast stroke is the best swimming stroke for the patient, with front and back crawl also being useful.

LATER EXERCISES

1. ½ gr. ½ st; (float on F) 1Hip and K straighten and bend.
2. pr. ly; (holding float) breast stroke leg movement.
3. sitt; (flipper on 1F) 1K straighten and bend.
4. Toe sup. ly; Hip and K bend and stretch.
5. fl. sup. ly; (flipper on F) 1Hip extend, abduct and medially rotate w. K extension.
6. ½ sup. ly; (flipper on 1F) 1L press d. and raise slowly
7. ½ sup. s. ly; (flipper on 1F) bicycling action quickly.
8. st; walking with long steps.
9. gr. pr. ly; Hip and K bend to chest and straighten.
10. step st; 1Hip and K straighten and bend.

FRACTURED SHAFTS OF TIBIA AND FIBULA

Normally the patient is fixed in a full-length plaster from the metatarsophalangeal joints of the toes to the thigh for 8–12 weeks. In some cases the bones may be plated and the plaster may be on for a shorter period of time. As the period of fixation is so long there is limitation of movement in the knee, ankle and subtaloid joints with weakness of all the muscles of the lower limb.

The pool is beneficial in mobilizing the joints of the lower limb. The muscles can be strengthened effectively by using buoyancy and patterned movements. The patient may limp owing to the muscle weakness and joint stiffness, but during re-education of walking buoyancy will assist the 'push off' and knee flexion.

When the plaster is removed the skin will be in a poor condition and loose scales should be removed before the patient enters the pool. The warmth of the water will improve the circulation to the skin and will therefore improve its nutrition. Water also has a drying effect and so the skin should be oiled after treatment.

EXERCISES

1. $\frac{1}{2}$ sup. ly; (float under knee) 1K straighten. Buoyancy assists the lower leg movement and the float encourages inner range quadriceps contraction.
2. fl. ly; stabilizations to knee.
3. sitt; 1K straighten and bend.
4. $\frac{1}{2}$ gr. st; 1Hip and K bend u. and d.
5. rch. gr. st; Hl. raise and lower.
6. $\frac{1}{2}$ sup. s. ly; 1K bend and straighten.
7. $\frac{1}{2}$ gr. wlk. st; (affected F behind) wt. transfer back F to front F (practise push off).
8. $\frac{1}{2}$ gr. wlk. st; (affected F behind) wt. transfer to fwd. F and practise K flex of affected L.
9. $\frac{1}{2}$ gr. wlk. st; (affected F forward) wt. transfer to fwd. F. Practise wt. bearing on affected L with straight K.
10. gr. step st; 1Hip and K straighten and bend (progress to shallower water).

Passive patella movements
Following immobilization, the patella femoral joint may be stiff; oscillatory passive movements may be used to mobilize this joint with the patient in $\frac{1}{2}$ sup. ly.

Progression is made to buoyancy resisted exercises and further progression by the addition of floats and flippers.

At the same time the patient should have exercises on land for the joints of the foot and be taught exercises to do at home.

FRACTURES ROUND THE KNEE JOINT

Supracondylar and condylar fractures of the femur, fractures of the patella and fractures of the tibial condyles may be treated in the pool.

Supracondylar fractures of the femur may be treated in the pool from four to seven weeks after the injury; treatment for fractures of the tibial condyles may begin in one or two weeks after the injury. With fractures of the patella the period of immobilization varies from 2–6 weeks depending on the type of fracture and the method of treatment.

In all the above fractures the quadriceps muscle will be weak and the knee joint movement limited. Treatment is similar to that described for fractures of the shafts of tibia and fibula. A quadriceps lag is, however, more likely to occur following these injuries. The patient is placed in the buoyancy-assisting or buoyancy-counterbalanced positions to treat this lag and the patient finds it easier than on land in side lying as the water supports the limb.

Injury to the common peroneal nerve may occur in fractures of the tibial condyles or in supracondylar fractures of the femur, resulting in a dropped foot. This is treated following similar principles to those applicable to other peripheral nerve lesions and as such are better treated on land.

Passive stretching to the tendo Achilles is of value when the patient is in the pool and it is unwise to have the patient walking in the water until the muscles show signs of recovery.

FRACTURES OF BONES OF THE FOOT

Fractures and dislocations round the ankle and foot are, on the whole, better treated on land than in the pool. Fractures of the calcaneum, particularly when bilateral, may be treated in the pool after about 3–4 weeks for re-education in walking. If gravitational oedema is a complication, the lateral pressure of the water will minimize this during walking practice. Patients with these fractures find walking in the pool less painful than walking on land and so their walking pattern is more normal.

FRACTURES ROUND THE SHOULDER JOINT

Pool therapy is valuable for patients sustaining such injuries as many of them are elderly and are disinclined to move the arm, holding it rigidly to the side with the shoulder girdle elevated. As soon as mobilization is allowed, active exercises are performed to regain shoulder and elbow movements and to strengthen the deltoid and shoulder girdle muscles. The warmth of the water reduces pain and buoyancy assists movement, and therefore it is easier to avoid or correct reversed humeroscapular rhythm, so that trick movements shall not develop.

In the later stages of treatment, provided that it is suitable for the patient, swimming can be introduced, the arm movements of both breast stroke and crawl being excellent for regaining shoulder movements.

Fractures and dislocations in the elderly. The elderly may suffer an impacted fracture of the neck of the humerus or a dislocated shoulder. In both instances pool treatment can begin in two to three days after the injury. As the fracture is so recent oedema and bruising will be present, making movement painful. Reassurance and encouragement should be given and care taken to avoid unguarded movements. The physiotherapist walks in front of the patient as he enters the pool and supports the arm, which will be in a sling. At first the patient sits on a high stool to limit the effects of buoyancy, but as treatment progresses the height of the stool is lowered and the sling discarded.

Hand, elbow and all shoulder movements are given, except that lateral rotation of the shoulder in abduction may be delayed for one to two weeks with a dislocated shoulder. At first the patient is in the sitting position and is given 'hold–relax' techniques to increase abduction and flexion of the shoulder, stabilizations to the shoulder joint and buoyancy-assisted exercises for the deltoid muscle. Progression is made to exercises with buoyancy counterbalanced in float support lying and finally to buoyancy-resisted exercises. As the muscle power improves floats are added to give a further progression. The breast stroke arm action may be done, sitting at first, and then progressing to doing it while walking through the water.

Great care is necessary with these patients as they are elderly and have the use of only one arm. This often appears to make them more nervous than patients with leg injuries.

EXERCISES
1. sitt; Sh. push u, push d. and relax.
2. sitt; Sh. pull f., push b. and relax.
3. sitt; H turn s. to s. (keeping sh. level).
4. sitt; 1A raise f. and lower.
5. sitt; 1A raise s. and lower.
6. rt. L bd. sitt; Fra turn i. and o.
7. rch. sitt; A carry s. and return.
8. bd. sitt; A stretch f. and bend; A stretch s. and bend.
9. rt. L bd. sitt; Fing. bend and stretch with wrist bend and stretch.

10. fl. ly; A push d. and return (hold sh. girdle in retraction).
11. fl. ly; A raise s. and return.
12. Hnd. sup. sitt; Elb. straighten to raise pelvis off seat.

PATTERNS

Suitable arm patterns are bilateral flexion, abduction and lateral rotation, single-arm abduction (modified in the presence of pain), flexion, abduction and lateral rotation in pr. ly. (advanced) and flexion, adduction and lateral rotation in pr. ly.

Isometric patterns may be used in the early stages; for example, bilateral arm abduction (Chapter 7).

Fractures and dislocations in the young. Younger patients suffer from unimpacted fractures of the surgical neck of the humerus or from dislocation of the shoulder. They have a longer period of immobilization and so pool therapy is delayed. For dislocations, pool treatment begins after approximately three weeks, and following an unimpacted fracture of the surgical neck of the humerus not for six to seven weeks. The scheme of treatment is similar to that for the elderly patient but progression is quicker.

Final exercises are stronger and will include swimming, especially back crawl. The final arm exercises that are given are similar to those given the patient with paraplegia (page 137).

FRACTURED SHAFT OF HUMERUS

This fracture occurs in a younger age group than that associated with fractures of the neck. The period of immobilization is usually 6–8 weeks and stiffness of the elbow and frequently of the shoulder joints result. Shoulder movements can usually be performed while the plaster is still on, and so it tends to become less stiff. Treatment is usually given on land only, but pool treatment is indicated if the elbow (or shoulder) remains stiff. If this is so, repeated contractions and 'hold–relax' techniques are given in the buoyancy-counterbalanced position.

EXERCISES

In addition the following exercises may be given:

1. sitt; breast stroke arm action.
2. acr. bd. sitt; Elb. stretch and bend.

3. str. gr. pr. ly; Elb. bend and stretch.
   Exercises 1–3 may be progressed by the addition of floats or bats.
4. gr. incl. pr. st; Elb. straighten and bend.
5. ½ gr. incl. tow. s. st; 1 Elb. stretch and bend.
6. swimming; breast stroke and crawl improve elbow and shoulder movement.

PATTERNS OF MOVEMENT

Patterns and shoulder exercises for these patients should be selected from those given above for fractures round the shoulder joint.

If the radial nerve is involved a dropped wrist will result and is treated on land.

If internal fixation is used, mobilization will begin at an earlier date and these patients do not usually require pool therapy.

FRACTURES OF THE SPINE

Conservative treatment of fractures of the spine involves a period of rest, and later exercises to increase the strength of the back extensor and abdominal muscles. At first pool exercises for the back extensor muscles are given and as the pain subsides flexion exercises are added. Exercises to work the back extensor muscles are performed isotonically but the trunk flexors are worked isometrically.

INITIAL EXERCISES

1. ½ sup. ly; alt. L push d.
2. ½ sup. incl. pr. ly; L raise.
3. ½ sup. ly; L swing from s. to s.
4. ½ sup. ly; L part and close.
5. ½ sup. s. ly; L swing b.
6. fl. sup. ly; A push d.
7. fl. sup. ly; (float under Buttocks) push Buttocks d. into float. Breast stroke swimming can be given.

Patterns

In the early stages, bilateral arm and leg patterns are suitable because the spinal muscles are working statically. For example, the bilateral leg abduction and the bilateral flexion, abduction and lateral rotation arm patterns may be used. Then bilateral arm extension may be added, and as muscle spasm subsides relaxation may be encouraged by using the trunk side-flexion pattern passively with the therapist fixing on the thorax.

LATER EXERCISES

As soon as flexion is allowed the following exercises may be added:

1. ½ sup. s. ly; Hip and knee bend f. and stretch b.
2. sitt; T turn from s. to s.
3. Toe sup. ly; double A back crawl.
4. sitt; K bend u.
5. incl. pr. ½ sup. st; Hip and K bend f. under stretcher and b.

Progress to:

6. str. gr. ½ sup. pr. ly; Hip and K bend f. and stretch b.

As the pain subsides and muscle power and joint mobility increases stronger exercises can be given:

7. ½ sup. ly; (float on Foot) L push d.
8. ½ sup. ly; 1L swing over opposite L and back.
9. fl. sup. ly; (float on Hand) A push d.
10. str. gr. ½ sup. pr. ly; (float on Foot) Hip and K bend f. and stretch b.
11. hve. gr. ly; (float on Foot) push Buttocks into water with K bend under.

Patterns

Suitable patterns are trunk side-flexion (*a*) with lower trunk moving and (*b*) with upper trunk moving. Flexion and extension trunk patterns are useful to work the trunk muscles isometrically and isotonically. Then the trunk flexion or extension with rotation patterns may be used.

Swimming should be encouraged. All strokes provide good work for the trunk muscles and help to increase their power. Back stroke and crawl are particularly good for extension, butterfly adds flexion, and trunk rotation is achieved during the arm movements of front or back crawl.

Fractures of the spine and transverse processes of the vertebrae will be treated earlier and will recover more quickly than compression fractures of the vertebral bodies.

In fracture–dislocation of the spine the spinal cord may be

injured, in which case the treatment is as for paraplegia. If the spinal cord has escaped injury, the fracture is reduced and the period of immobilization is approximately 12 weeks. The treatment is similar to that for a compression fracture but the progress will be slower.

SURGERY FOR THE SPINE

Various surgical procedures may be performed on the spine. These include 'fenestration' which is an excision of the ligamentum flavum and little, if any, of the adjacent laminae; hemilaminectomy, or laminectomy, which is removal of one or both laminae; fusion of the spine.

After fenestration or laminectomy, pool therapy can begin as soon as the sutures are out—approximately 12 days after the operation. The aims of treatment will be to relieve pain in the back and aid relaxation; to strengthen the extensor muscles of the back and the abdominal muscles; to increase the mobility of all movements of the lumbar spine, especially flexion; and to restore the patient's confidence in his back and to reinforce posture sense, back care and lifting.

If the surgeon advocates a flexion-oriented programme for the patient then flexion must remain as the main theme of pool treatment. Otherwise, exercises may be selected from the following examples.

EASY EXERCISES
1. fl. sup. ly; conscious relaxation.
2. fl. sup. ly; L swing from s. to s. (Fig. 10.1).
3. $\frac{1}{2}$ sup. ly; (K bend) K roll from s. to s.
4. $\frac{1}{2}$ sup. ly; alt. L push d. and u.
5. $\frac{1}{2}$ sup. std. ly; 1L push d. and u., 1L lift u. and over (as L cross, spine is rotated).
6. $\frac{1}{2}$ sup. pr. ly; L bend u. under $\frac{1}{2}$ stretcher with static hold at limit of range.
7. B. sup. st; hold–relax to hamstrings to gain straight leg raising.
8. hve. gr. st; (at rail) K bend u. or sitt.—K bend u. (Fig. 10.2).
9. $\frac{1}{2}$ sup. s. ly; Hip and K bend u. and stretch b.
10. walking.

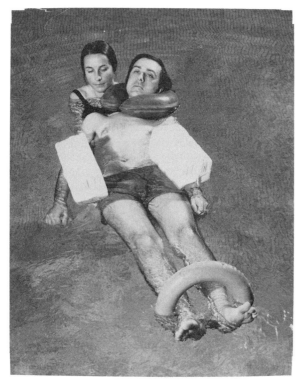

Fig. 10.1. Trunk side-flexion pattern; 10 days post-laminectomy.

LATER EXERCISES

As mobility and power improve the following exercises may be given:

1. $\frac{1}{2}$ sup. s. ly; (floats on F)—L push d. (repeat on other s.).
2. $\frac{1}{2}$ sup. pr. ly; L bend d. and u. under stretcher and stretch b.
3. sitt; hold–relax to B extensors.

The hold is applied by the therapist's forearm on the posterior aspect of the patient's thighs; buoyancy assists into the new range following the relaxation phase.

4. walking with large steps.
5. walking backwards.
6. swimming; backstroke progress to breast stroke.

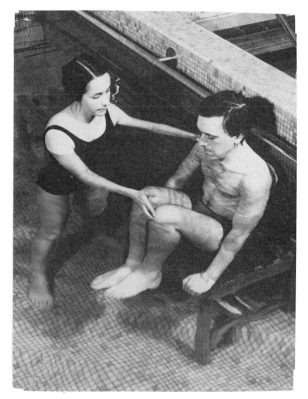

Fig. 10.2. Buoyancy assisting flexion of the lumbar spine. Same patient as in Fig. 10.1.

7. hve. gr. ly; (float on F) Pelvis push down with K bend.
8. gr. std. st; (bat in Hnd) T turn from s. to s. or gr. sitt; (bat in Hnd) T turn from s. to s. (Fig. 10.3).
9. fl. sup. ly; (float on F) L push d.
10. Toe sup. ly; T bend s. to s.
11. walking, changing direction to commands.

The Bad Ragaz techniques, as described in Chapter 7, for flexion and extension and side flexion patterns, can be given within the limits of pain from the beginning of treatment. If the back is too painful for these patterns those for the arm and leg may be given initially.

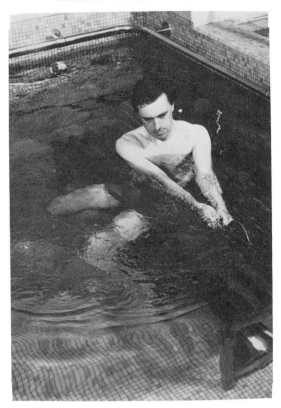

Fig. 10.3. Rotation of the thoracic spine. Same patient as in Figs 10.1 and 10.2.

Spinal fusion
Following this operation patients are in bed for approximately 4 weeks. They are taught back care and are discharged home. After a further 12 weeks, mobilizing and strengthening exercises are taught. Pool therapy is indicated if the patient does not regain movement satisfactorily and he would follow the regime described above. As these patients tend to be young, complications are uncommon.

All patients who have had back surgery are encouraged to take up swimming as regular recreation.

SURGERY FOR THE PELVIS

Hemipelvectomy. In this operation the sacro-iliac and symphysis pubis joints are divided and the hip bone is removed. Patients begin pool treatment when the wound has healed, in approximately 2 weeks. Partial weight-bearing walking with elbow crutches may begin 10 days after the operation.

Pool therapy is used to gain hip and knee movements (Fig. 10.4) and to help in regaining a normal walking pattern.

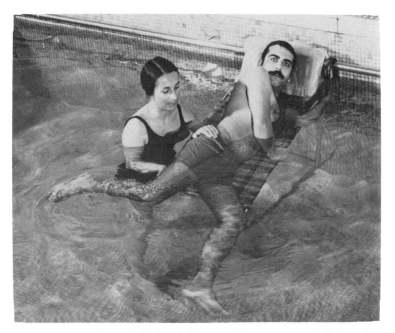

Fig. 10.4. Extension of the hip joint 3 weeks post-operatively showing range of hip extension.

The lack of bony attachments for the muscles makes for difficulties in both phases of walking. When the affected leg is in the stance phase, it is difficult to swing the other leg through because there is no hip abductor action to counterbalance the hip bone on the swinging side (Fig. 10.5). When the affected leg is in the swing phase, it is difficult to lift up the soft tissues in order to flex the hip and knee, so the patient tends to thrust the trunk to the weight

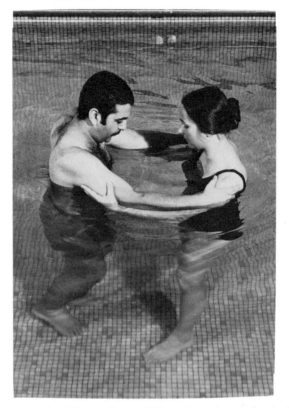

Fig. 10.5. Assisted walking in the pool. Note therapist standing in front of patient.

bearing side to lift the foot of the affected leg off the ground.

With practice, using buoyancy to assist hip hitching, these patients attain a walking pattern which is remarkably normal, even on land.

SURGERY FOR THE HIP

With the exception of arthrodesis, all types of hip surgery aim to provide a mobile, pain-free hip and to construct a suitable weight-bearing joint. Surgery may follow trauma or may be used for osteoarthritis of the hip. There are a variety of procedures that can be used and the choice rests with the surgeon.

Arthroplasty. The patient is usually middle aged or elderly. Various procedures using different forms of prosthesis may be carried out. Excision arthroplasty (Girdlestone's pseudo-arthrosis) is used where another form of arthroplasty has not been a success or where this is the only form of operation possible. After total hip replacement the patient is up in 2–5 days and is discharged home with sticks or crutches, having been taught exercises to practise. Pool therapy would be indicated prior to discharge, after the stitches had been removed, if the patient had unacceptable stiffness of the joint, weakness of muscles or difficulty with walking. Sometimes patients are referred for pool therapy, after discharge when progression to full rehabilitation is too slow in the opinion of the surgeon. Suitable exercises are as indicated for fractures of the neck of the femur, with the same precautions relating to the application of resistance (page 155).

Following an excision arthroplasty a period of traction is required and the treatment is similar to that for a fractured neck of femur. Owing to the instability of the joint more of these patients require pool treatment.

SURGERY FOR THE KNEE

With the exception of arthrodesis, surgery to the knee results in two main problems—joint stiffness and quadriceps weakness. Treatment is therefore aimed at regaining quadriceps power and knee mobility. Owing to the weight-bearing nature of the joint it is important to have a treatment programme that progresses by reducing the time in the pool and increasing the time in the gymnasium.

Synovectomy. Following synovectomy of the knee, treatment in the pool may begin approximately 10 days after the operation. The value of pool treatment is twofold: there can be a fine grading of quadriceps exercises and, as the operation is frequently performed for rheumatoid arthritis, other joints and muscles can be treated at the same time.

Patellectomy. This operation may be performed for osteoarthritis or following a fracture of the patella. Postoperatively the knee may be immobilized for 2 weeks for osteoarthritis and 2–6 weeks following a fracture as the extensor mechanism has been sutured. Once movement is permitted pool therapy may begin. This is a valuable method for regaining knee flexion. Many of these patients are young and advanced exercises should be included in the final stages of treatment.

Menisectomy. Pool treatment is usually only necessary if rehabilitation is complicated by extreme pain, muscle weakness and joint stiffness. Treatment can begin as soon as sutures are out. In this instance only a few treatments are required.

Arthroplasty. As with the hip, there are various forms of arthroplasty, the most common being the Attenborough, the Geo-Medic and the Stanmore Hinge. When a hinge prosthesis is used, no more than 90° knee flexion can be regained. Pool treatment may begin after removal of the sutures, approximately 12 days from the operation. Knee flexion will have been minimal (approx. 30°) up to this point; therefore it is important to emphasize this movement in pool treatment. As a general rule, patients are not discharged from hospital until knee flexion is at least 60°. The weight-bearing walking pattern can be re-educated early in the pool and this gives the patient confidence in the new joint. Partial weight-bearing walking may begin on land 4–5 days after the operation, provided that there is no quadriceps lag on straight leg raising.

Quadricepsplasty. The value of pool therapy after this operation is the fine grading of quadriceps strengthening and the correction of quadriceps lag. A combined programme of dry-land and pool therapy often gives the best results.

Surgical repair of knee ligaments

Lateral ligament instability. In a MacIntosh repair, the fascia lata is used to reinforce the lateral ligament. The knee is immobilized in a plaster extending from groin to metatarsal heads in 30° flexion for 6 weeks.

Medial ligament instability. A pes anserinus operation involves the re-siting of the insertion of gracilis and sartorius forwards and upwards.

The knee is immobilized in a full-length plaster, in flexion, at an angle of 90–60° for 6 weeks.

Suturing of ruptured medial and lateral ligaments. Following suturing of medial and lateral ligaments the knee is usually immobilized in a plaster cylinder for 6 weeks with the knee in a few degrees short of extension.

After cruciate repair, the period of immobilization is usually 3–4 weeks. Fixation is a plaster cylinder with the knee in full extension.

Following these operations, pool therapy is very useful from the day of removal of the plaster. The aims are to strengthen the quadriceps using finely graded progressions, to prevent quadriceps lag, to regain movement of the knee, and to rehabilitate the limb as a functional unit.

Special points
Knee flexion should not be forced beyond 90° for several weeks after a repair of ruptured ligaments.

After MacIntosh or pes anserinus repair, treatment should emphasize inner-range work for the quadriceps.

The patient's confidence in the limb may be restored by walking in the pool and by standing in turbulent water, turbulence being created first by the physiotherapist and then by the patient using bats. Swimming, especially breast stroke, is beneficial in mobilizing and restoring confidence.

INITIAL EXERCISES
A selection of the following exercises would be suitable for these patients:

1. sitt; 1K straighten and bend.
2. ½ sup. ly; (float under 1K) 1K straighten (buoyancy assists lower-leg movement and the float encourages inner-range quadriceps contraction) (Fig. 10.6).
3. ½ sup. s. ly; (manual support on thigh) 1K bend and stretch (Fig. 10.7).
4. ½ sup. s. ly; bicycling action.
5. gr. st; 1K bend and straighten.
6. gr. ½ st; 1Hip and K bend f. and stretch b.
7. ½ gr. ½ st; 1L swing f. and b.
8. sitt; ; alt. F. pull. u. and d.
9. fl. ly; stabilization of the knee muscles.
10. st; Hl. raise and lower.
11. sitt; stand up and sit d.
12. gr. st; mark time—encourage flex. of affected K (Fig. 10.8).
13. ½ sup. pr. ly; breast stroke leg action.

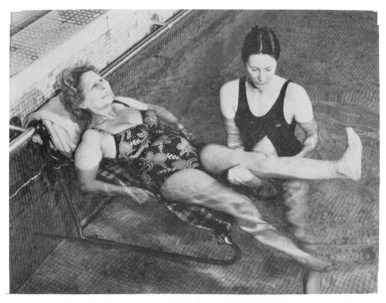

Fig. 10.6. Quadriceps contractions over rubber ring in a patient who has had repair of the medial ligament, left knee.

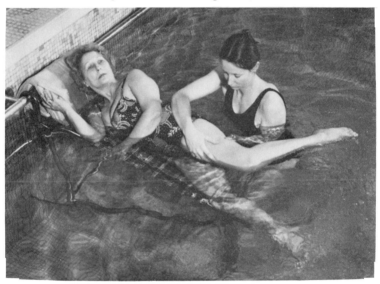

Fig. 10.7. Flexion of the knee joint in side lying. Same patient as in Fig. 10.6.

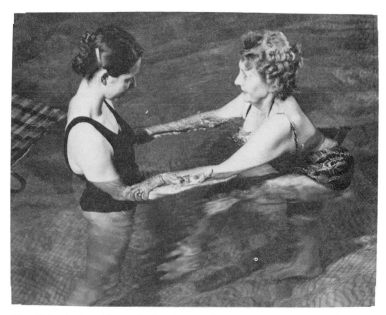

Fig. 10.8. Assisted knee flexion in standing. Same patient as in Figs 10.6 and 10.7.

14. walking practice—see Chapter 7 and the exercises under fractures of tibia and fibula.
These exercises may be progressed by the addition of floats or flippers.

LATER EXERCISES

1. Toe sup. ly; Hip and K bend and stretch (start with arms by side and progress to yd. position and then by holding bats in the hand).
2. step st; step u. and d.
3. breast stroke swimming.
4. walking with wide steps, and quickly.
5. walking backwards, forwards and sideways with turning to commands.
6. walking through turbulent water.
7. gr. $\frac{1}{2}$ sup. pr. ly; K bend under stretcher and stretch b.

Patterns
Isotonic patterns incorporating knee flexion and extension are

suitable. Bilateral leg abduction pattern would help to strengthen quadriceps.

Scales prosthesis
These are made-to-measure prostheses, for the lower end of the femur or the upper end of the tibia. Pool therapy may begin when the sutures are removed. Emphasis is placed on quadriceps strengthening and walking re-education. Resisted knee flexion should be avoided for 8 weeks and knee flexion should not be beyond 90° for 12 weeks.

SURGERY FOR THE SHOULDER

Surgery for the shoulder joint may be necessary following recurrent dislocation or fractures.

Recurrent dislocation. The aim of surgery is to secure the head of the humerus and to approximate its articular surface with the glenoid cavity. Fixation is usually for 4–6 weeks, with the arm by the side to avoid abduction and rotation. Mobilization in the pool is started as soon as possible after the fixation is removed. Re-education is started with the patient sitting on a stool so that the physiotherapist can see every direction of movement and can control any tendency to reversed scapulohumeral rhythm. Otherwise the treatment is similar to that for a young patient with a fractured neck of humerus, except that combined abduction and lateral rotation should never be forced. If using the flexion, abduction and lateral rotation pattern, one hand should be placed on the scapula and one hand on the patient's hand to control the amount of abduction and lateral rotation gained.

Swimming is useful for regaining mobility, but care is necessary because of the need to avoid abduction and lateral rotation. Breast stroke and then front crawl can be used in the later stages, but back crawl should be avoided.

SURGERY FOR THE ELBOW

Excision arthroplasty (removal of the head of the radius). Arthroplasty may be required after a compound fracture or fracture–dislocation of the elbow. Movement of the elbow and radio-ulnar joints is allowed in 10–14 days after surgery. Stiffness is not a complication, so emphasis is on strengthening biceps and triceps. Instability of the joint is likely to follow arthroplasty unless adequate muscle control is regained, and at the same time elbow joint movement must never be forced.

EXERCISES

Sitting is a suitable starting position for early exercises as buoyancy is counterbalanced. The following are examples of suitable exercises:

1. rch. sitt; (palms d.) Elb. bend and stretch.

Progress to:

2. rch. sitt; (bat parallel to surface of water) Elb. bend and stretch.

Progress to:

3. turning bat broadside through the water.
4. sitt; breast stroke A action.
5. ½ yd. gr. ly; alt. L push d. and u. (stabilizing for elbow).

Progress to:

6. str. gr. fl. sup. pr. ly; Elb. bend and stretch.
7. gr. sitt; Buttocks lift off stool.
8. rch. gr. incl. away st; Elb. bend and stretch, with T pull f. and push b.

SOFT-TISSUE INJURIES

LIMBS

There is very little indication for pool therapy for soft-tissue injuries of the limbs except for partial rupture of the ligaments of the knee joint. These injuries may be treated by immobilization until healing is complete and pool therapy will be similar to that given following surgical repair for a complete rupture.

THE SPINE

Ligamentous injuries. Initially strains, partial or complete rupture of the ligaments of the back, are usually treated by rest. Movement is allowed when the pain has decreased. Pool therapy can be of value to relax muscle spasm and to regain movement, but some patients, who are unaccustomed to water, are unable to relax, with subsequent increase in pain and in muscle spasm of the back extensors. This group may benefit from pool therapy after treatment on land aimed at encouraging movement and relaxation.

On the first day of pool therapy it is often valuable to have the patient in head support lying; the physiotherapist grasps the patient's thorax and walks backwards, moving him gently from side to side. The patient is then encouraged to do active movements. Thereafter the treatment follows the regime given for a fractured spine on page 112. It is important that the patient is taught on land how to prevent further injury to his back.

INTERVERTEBRAL DISC LESIONS

Lumbar region. The nuclear protrusion with the ruptured-annulus type of lesion benefits from a combination of mobilizations on land and pool therapy. The patient usually has a period of bed rest from 2 to 6 weeks from the onset of pain. Following this he will have stiffness of the spine and the nerve roots or trunk of the sciatic nerve may be bound down by adhesions, resulting in unilateral limitation of straight leg raising. Such a patient responds well to a regime of daily mobilizations for 1–2 weeks, aimed at freeing the nerve and mobilizing the stiff segments of the spine. Pool therapy is started in the second week, aimed at strengthening the back extensor and abdominal muscles and at mobilizing the lumbar spine. Exercises for mobilizing should start in positions where the upper trunk is fixed and the pelvis is moving; only when the stiff segments are free should larger range movements of the whole spine be included.

Patients with other disc lesions. These present a widely varying pattern of clinical signs and symptoms. Following careful examination the principles of mobilizing, strengthening and stabilizing are applied.

As indicated above, pool therapy is of value in regaining mobility, provided there is localized mobilizing of stiff segments, first on land, and then in the pool. Exercises are localized to the lumbar spine before total spinal movements are given. Equal importance is given to strengthening the back extensor muscles and the abdominal muscles and both groups can be worked against buoyancy. Where the main problem is instability this is probably treated more effectively on land.

Thoracic spine. Pool therapy is rarely indicated for thoracic disc lesions. Scheuermann's vertebral osteochondritis is a condition involving changes in the thoracic discs and vertebrae and occurs in the 13–16 age group. These patients suffer from thoracic pain and stiffness, which responds well to all forms of swimming and exercises for the extensor muscles of the spine. If the condition is severe, the patient has to rest on a plaster bed, but when mobilization is allowed pool therapy provides a stimulus to the patient's morale.

11

Water Activity Based on the Halliwick Method

Children and adults who are handicapped need not be denied the delights of movement. Physical activity on land may be hard for such people but in the water they come into their own. Most people enjoy the water and want to learn to swim; and the sense of achievement when they master the art is enormous. They gain confidence, their self-respect is enhanced and they acquire a social benefit, for in the water they can compete with their normal counterparts. Handicapped people, like others, benefit from incentives to improve their stamina and technique; therefore, the effects are both psychological and physical.

A child must experience active movement if he is to develop, and lack of physical experience may well be a major factor in the slow development of the handicapped child. Activity in water is a means of widening his experience.

Water as a medium for activity has both therapeutic and recreational aspects. Where these aspects are based on the same method they become complimentary to each other, and a programme of continual rehabilitation, through properly thought out recreation, can be promoted. Recreationally, larger patterns of movements are involved, whilst therapeutically such patterns can be refined.

Where children are concerned such an approach is invaluable. Hydrotherapy, in the strictly accepted sense of being purely remedial, is not of great value; at the same time purely recreational programmes directed towards the teaching of swimming by normal methods do not always succeed because allowances for the disability are not made or the handicap is misunderstood.

Water offers the experience of finding one's body acted upon by two principal forces—gravity or downthrust, buoyancy or upthrust. It provides the potential of exercise in three dimensions which cannot be achieved on land. There is massive stimulation for perceptual training visually, aurally and through the skin receptors, owing to the effects of turbulence, heat and hydrostatic pressure. There is also improved respiration, balance control and rotational control, which are critical in water owing to buoyancy and metacentric effects, and psychological effects.

If a child is asked whether he would like to play about in the water he would most probably reply, 'Yes'; therefore any programme of exercise would be hidden by playing. This can be given a positive aspect if the programme is designed to include the teaching of swimming with the remedial exercises.

A definite approach now emerges, as few children, however timorous, can resist joining in with those happily at play. It is essential that the child or adult is mentally happy in the water as well as being physically adjusted, so that the most beneficial atmosphere can be created; then demands for greater activity are likely to be met. Mental adjustment cannot be obtained simply by assurance on the part of the therapist that 'everything will be all right'—it can only come from within the person who has become completely balanced in an element which is naturally strange to him.

As creatures of land, we make subsconscious adaptations to the effects of gravity which are virtually useless in water and result in gross postural confusion. Many are apprehensive and tense in water, and the handicapped person will have other and specific inhibitions which arise as a result of his physical disability. He may suffer, for example, from a very acute fear of falling, difficulty in communication, inability to move readily or at will, inability to control sporadic or unwanted movement, poor or badly controlled respiration, lack of comprehension and asymmetry of shape and density.

To achieve mental adjustment and self-assurance, an understanding of water—continual adjustment to its feel, its turbulence, its buoyancy and its weight, especially where these may affect the body balance—is vitally important. Correct breathing control should be repeatedly emphasized; likewise the ability to recover to a safe breathing position. This can be obtained through games and activities that are fun, and at the same time encourage subtle control of the body.

In all programmes of activity the fullest range of sensation and movement should be used—change of pace, change of position, change of atmosphere from seriousness to laughter. Water is critical of shape and density. Everyone has a balance problem in water since none of us is completely symmetrical and our relative density varies. The handicapped person in whom shape and density are markedly altered has particular problems. It is possible by studying the shape and density of the person going into the water to predict what will happen, and to give instructions as to the actions that can be taken to counteract any rotational effect due to the disability. These instructions may provide mental adjustment prior to entering the water, so that once in the water the person may perceive any rotational effect and take the necessary correcting action.

The importance of studying shape and density cannot be sufficiently stressed; this means observing the person anteriorly, posteriorly and laterally, from in front, from behind and from both sides. To observe the alterations in shape along the longitudinal axis of the body, the person can be supported supine in the water, the therapist standing at the person's head, support being given just below waist level, the centre of balance of the body (Fig. 11.1). From observation of shape and density the person's particular balance and rotational problems become evident and a programme of activity planned which encourages control of rotation, balance restoration and its maintenance.

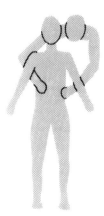

Fig. 11.1. Physiotherapist supporting patient.

Apart from the factors of shape and density the therapist must recognize the two extremes of posture in water. They may be described as 'stick' and 'ball' (Fig. 11.2). The body in the upright position standing on a relatively small area—the 'stick'—is disturbed easily, and when horizontal is readily rotated about its longitudinal axis. The rolled up position—the 'ball'—provides more stable balance and considerable effort is required to change the position of the body. Therefore, all early activities and exercises should be carried out in shapes that tend to be 'balled up'. As balance and control develop these shapes should be unrolled to be longer, thus requiring a greater degree of control.

Shape can be altered deliberately by the handicapped person himself through movement of the body or a body part; the alteration may occur owing to involuntary movement, or owing to the active intervention of the therapist. Additionally, tension can alter shape and tension can be created by actions such as 'gripping', 'holding the breath' or 'shutting the eyes'. Negative phrases, such as these and 'sinking' and 'drowning', should *never* be used. A positive approach should be developed. Such phrases as 'lying in bed', 'head on pillow', 'rolling over', 'sitting in your chair', 'hands on the table', are associated with land habits and safety and aid mental adjustment.

Exercises and activities should be constructed on the following lines: (*a*) a primary activity in which the person is shown and, if necessary, assisted in the creation of a movement or a shape; (*b*) a follow-up activity requiring the creation of the movement or shape against the effect and weight of moving water; and (*c*) an oblique activity which may suggest a different objective but still contains the primary activity—the movement is then observed to ensure that it can be produced when required, without prompting. Examples of activities are given at the end of this chapter.

We have seen that the aims of the activities are to encourage the acquisition of confidence, to understand, enjoy and be safe in water, to breathe well and, ultimately, to swim. The programme of activities is planned along the following lines and, throughout, the person should be encouraged to treat the pool in as normal a manner as possible, that is to say as a medium to improve and extend his patterns of posture, movement and independence.

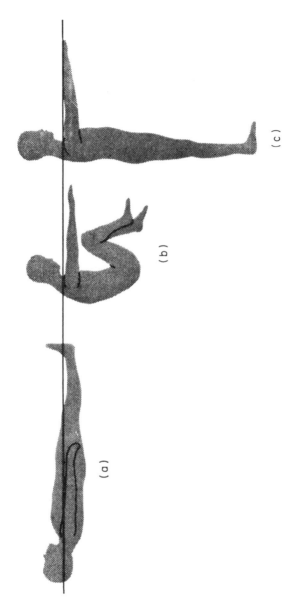

Fig. 11.2. (a) 'stick'; (b) 'ball'; (c) 'stick'.

ENTRY AND EXIT

When first introducing children to the water it is advisable to break up the surface with floating objects, as an expanse of water can seem vast and frightening, especially to the very young: the height of the bath edge from the waterline and the surface area of the water, viewed at eye level, will seem enormous to a child. Therefore, care should be taken to shield the child from positions that accentuate height and distance. For instance, short-distance focal points can be achieved by working across the shortest distance of the pool, by facing into a corner, or by allowing interesting objects to float on the water within sight of the child.

A method of entry and exit over the side of the bath that the child can manage for himself in due course is advisable, for he may not always swim in a pool where steps or a ramp and help are available to get him in and out of the water. In addition, he becomes independent, helping his self-confidence, self-esteem and normalizing his existence.

In some cases adults may also demonstrate anxieties about entering the water for the first time, and the therapist should always precede the person into the water and give the same attention to details of entry as expressed above for the child.

Independent entry and exit for adults over the side is frequently possible, but in some instances, especially with the very elderly, alternative methods of entry and exit may have to be used. Wherever possible, however, mobility and independence should be encouraged.

ENTRY

The therapist should always get into the water first and stand ready to receive the child. She should enter quietly, causing as little splash as possible, and ensure that she immerses her shoulders, and blows bubbles in the water. Such actions reassure the child.

The child sitting on the side is encouraged to put his hands forwards on the therapist's shoulders, his feet free of the wall; he is now in a 'ball' shape. The therapist's hands are placed under his arms, around his back and just below his scapulae [Fig. 11.3(1)]. The therapist should talk to him, encouraging him to blow as he comes towards the water [Fig. 11.3(2)].

Once in, immediately proceed to an activity such as jumping,

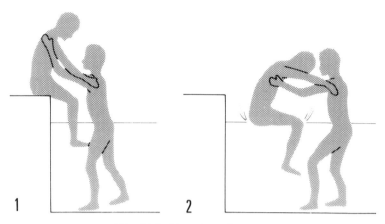

Fig. 11.3. Entry into the water.

allowing no time for anxious thoughts. Jumping also teaches breathing and head control and is a prerequisite for independence. The progression of entry is to 'hands on hands' (Fig. 11.4) then allowing a gap between the therapist's hands and the child's (Fig. 11.5). The forward action of entry must be facilitated and become automatic, extension being avoided at all times.

EXIT

Exit over the side should be developed in such a manner that the child's independence is aided. This involves the child placing his

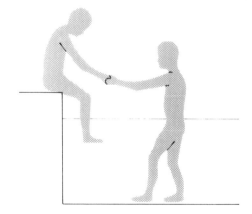

Fig. 11.4. Hands on hands.

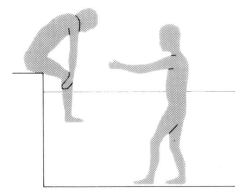

Fig. 11.5. Gap between therapist's and child's hands.

hands on the wall and, with assistance from the therapist holding both hips just below the greater trochanter, achieving a position lying on the wall, with the legs straight down the side of the pool [Fig. 11.6 (1 and 2)]. He then 'wriggles' forward pushing on his hands [Fig. 11.6(3)]. His legs should be lifted high and clear of the water as he moves forward until his hips are well over the side of the pool. He is assisted to roll over and sit up [Fig. 11.6 (4 and 5)].

Care must be taken where head control is limited and the exit modified to allow for flexor synergies of arms. In cases of spina bifida, if a urinary appliance is worn, the hip on the appliance side must be lifted well clear so that the appliance remains in situ.

HOLDS

The way in which the person is held in the water can affect the development of balance. The main object must always be to give the person the maximum feel of his own balanced position with the minimum of support. Whatever his body position he should be held near or opposite to the centre of balance of his body, at approximately his waistline, i.e. between T11 and S2. Although in the early stages the person may grip the therapist, this should be reduced eventually to a light hold, as gripping induces tension and destroys the sense of balance.

The therapist should remember always to adopt a position which enables the person to see and communicate easily without disturbing his balance unnecessarily. To achieve rapport with the

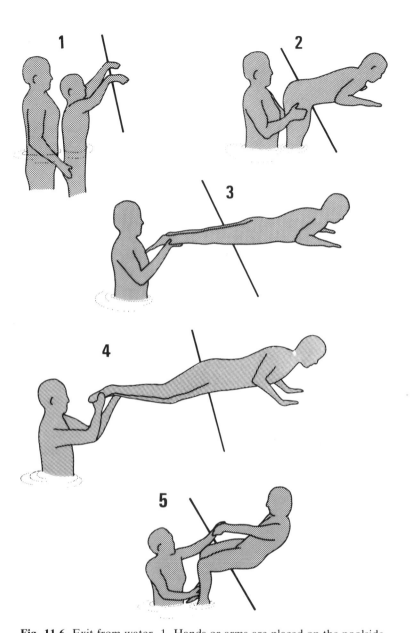

Fig. 11.6. Exit from water. 1. Hands or arms are placed on the poolside. 2. The therapist assists the forward movement on to the poolside. 3. The swimmer pushes on the hands to move forwards on the poolside; the therapist assists the swimmer to lift the legs high and clear of the water. 4. The rolling action is facilitated by the therapist when necessary. 5. Attaining the sitting position; the therapist gives assistance with the hands.

person it is vital that he has a feeling of closeness and can see the therapist at his own eye level, without having to turn unduly or extend his head in order to view her face.

BREATHING CONTROL

Holding the breath is a major factor in the creation of tension within the body. The development of a natural breathing rhythm is essential to anyone involved in activity in water; therefore, the person must be told to blow when the water is near his face and this must become an automatic skill.

The effect of blowing tends to bring the head forward, in contrast to the loss of control that follows the withdrawal or flinching action of the head when water is splashed on the face. Blowing should be in the background of all activities and should become an automatic skill, so that a good breathing rhythm is continually combined with other activities to ensure that the person is relaxed and balanced in water.

SAFETY AND RECOVERY

Safety and recovery are closely linked with the two planes of rotation in water—forward or vertical, turning or lateral. The person must be taught how to use his head to control the position of his body at all times, and to regain a safe breathing position.

Forward, or vertical, rotation is the ability to recover from a supine position to the vertical. It requires strong flexion of the whole body followed by exact balance of the head over the body to remain in a balanced vertical position.

Turning, or lateral, rotation requires control in both the vertical and horizontal planes. When lying the person must be able to control the axial rotation of his body which can occur either as a result of the asymmetry due to his handicap or because the movement of either the water or his body disturbs his position.

A combination of vertical and lateral rotation completes the person's ability to recover to a safe breathing position. If he should fall forwards in the water he should be instructed to turn his head in order to rotate his body until he is lying on his back. From there he can recover to the vertical and control is complete.

FLOTATION EQUIPMENT

The use of flotation equipment—except when a specific effect is required in remedial exercises—is highly undesirable and in some cases dangerous. Each handicapped person has a balance problem peculiar to himself, the effect of which can be altered completely or even reversed; it is also extremely difficult to adjust flotation equipment to ensure that the required balance position is maintained under any circumstance. The use of flotation equipment obviates one of the greatest advantages of working in the water, that of developing a fine degree of balance control. Owing to his handicap the person may well live in a world of appliances on land, but in water he can become completely independent and move in total freedom.

ACTIVITIES

The simple skills of standing, walking, jumping—both forwards and backwards—and turning in the water must be acquired as a basis for independence and to prepare the person for swimming. All activities should begin with the stable 'ball' position. As control improves the person can be encouraged to unroll his body into the 'stick' position to achieve more finely balanced movements.

Buoyancy as a force in water can be used to assist movement and counter gravitational effects. To understand about upthrust or buoyancy the person can be encouraged to push down on objects less dense than water—when released they will rise to the surface.

When the person is blowing into the water and has gained some rotational control, activities that take him to the bottom of the pool can be introduced. In the 'ball' shape the person will come to the surface quickly. In appreciating that water pushes him up to the surface, mental adjustment is almost complete. Such activities required good respiratory control, but the breath must *never* be held.

Plastics screwtop lids to jars sink slowly and it is great fun retrieving them at different depths; if they are of different colours and a certain number of points is awarded to each colour, then the activity becomes competitive and in a subtle manner increases mental adjustment—an activity especially suitable for children. Furthermore, to seek these objects the person must keep his eyes open under water—a skill vital to any swimmer.

It is at this stage, if not before, that the person will begin paddling himself about and he can progress to 'strokes' that are within his capabilities and related to his shape, density, control and mobility. There is no limit to the activities that can be devised. Objectives can be achieved through recreation but the therapist must bear in mind the teaching point of each activity so that its therapeutic and recreational content is carried through. Greater benefit is often derived from group treatment and the person gains from the companionship, competitiveness it offers, and is encouraged to work longer and concentrate harder.

REMEDIAL EXERCISES

Many of these may be incorporated in other activities.

As an example of an activity for a child which incorporates the specific movement of abduction of the hips, 'Hickory Dickory Dock' can be recited, since it combines the specific movement desired with learning about weight of water, body balance and awareness, head control and mental adjustment.

Purpose: to encourage disengagement.
Appreciation: body awareness and balance
Formation: swimmer stands facing the instructor (small children in deep water stand on the instructor's bent knees). The instructor holds the swimmer at the centre of balance of the body, i.e. at approximately waist level.
Instruction—sing 'Hickory Dickory Dock', 'ticking' like a clock from side to side to encourage abduction, lateral head control and appreciation of the weight of water. 'The mouse ran up the clock'—climb up the clock by climbing up the instructor, encouraging some disengagement and head and body control. 'The clock struck one'—clap hands over head encouraging further disengagement, arm movement, body awareness and head and body control. 'The mouse ran down'—run down the instructor and 'blow' the water, encouraging movement and forward head control and breathing. 'Hickory Dickory Dock'—repeat the 'ticking' movement.

As performance improves the instructor can give less help with balance and finally, to ensure lateral stability, can push the swimmer gently but firmly from side to side in the 'ticking' and see if he restores to the triangular position and is controlling his body forwards and backwards.

A triangular shape is one in which the swimmer's legs are widely parted sideways, the arms being close to the side of the body. If this shape is pushed sideways, water will restore it to the upright position, provided that the sideways movement is not too great.

Walking sideways, either in a circle or across the pool, will encourage increased abduction, head and trunk side-flexion in the adult. At the same time he will appreciate that water has weight, and the need for balance and head control. Mental adjustment is enhanced.

It should be remembered that in water buoyancy tends to minimize the effects of gravity, particularly when more than two-thirds of the body is immersed and when the body is floating. This means that there is not the same demand on the anti-gravity muscles, in addition to the other advantages.

CEREBRAL PALSY

Spasticity. The person with spasticity will find it easier to move because of the physiological effects, and if activities firstly of a swinging nature and later of a rotatory nature are introduced—all performed rhythmically—spasticity will be reduced.

Where head control is poor or does not exist the body can be held in a 'ball' shape and rocked gently forwards and backwards around the centre of buoyancy (Fig. 11.7). The rocking movements should be commensurate with the degree of head control—starting with a

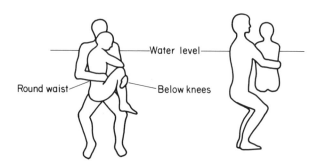

Fig. 11.7. Body held in 'ball' shape position.

minute movement away from the vertical in a forwards and backwards direction. As control improves so the swing can be increased.

In the hemiplegic person this position facilitates an extension pattern of the arm and a flexion pattern of the leg on the affected side. In the flaccid state protraction of the shoulder, and extension of the elbow, are obtained together with flexion at hip and knee. When tone is increased maintenance of this position combined with gentle rocking helps decrease tone. The therapist supports the person at the centre of balance around the waist and just below the knees and is able to facilitate and/or control the swing when necessary. By holding the person away from the therapist's body, many adverse responses may be avoided. In this position not only can the person's movements be observed, but facilitation and/or control more easily introduced when required.

Athetosis and ataxia. All involuntary movement will be damped down in water, and fine balance control can be taught in all positions by the use of turbulence appropriately placed and by activities that demand stability against turbulent effect.

When 'scissoring' occurs, lateral or rolling rotation should be taught early.

Care should be taken with persons suffering from cerebral palsy, especially in the early stages, to avoid the effects of extensor thrust of the head and neck under the water. In addition, before carrying out underwater activity a check should be made for any similar movement that could cause the mouth to be opened involuntarily.

SPINA BIFIDA

The need for consideration of shape and density is essential in children with spina bifida; both factors will be altered, and the less dense lower limbs will have a tendency to float high, whether the child is lying supine or prone in the water. Vertical rotation, or forward recovery, is, therefore, of vital importance to these children. An even greater degree of vertical rotational control is essential where hydrocephalus is a complicating factor. This applies also to paraplegia, polyneuritis and peripheral nerve lesions.

ATROPHIES

Such conditions will have altered shape and density and attention must be paid to where these alterations are and the programme planned accordingly. Forward and lateral rotational control are of great importance, and actions such as bringing the arms out of the water, thus introducing gravitational effects, may be necessary.

CONDITIONS CAUSING BODY ASYMMETRY
Some conditions, such as hemiplegia or unilateral amputations, cause asymmetry of the body shape, and it is important to develop lateral rotation in these instances.

ORTHOPAEDIC AND CONGENITAL CONDITIONS
Shape and density will be of importance in these conditions and the appropriate rotational control taught. Where joint range is to be increased, games that involve the whole body but lay emphasis on the joints that need exercising should be employed. For instance, the ability to regain the upright position from lying—vertical rotation—requires strong flexion of trunk, hips, knees and cervical spine with flexion of the shoulders in abduction. Thus a number of movements can be improved in this activity, which is of vital importance to the person in order that he can always regain a safe breathing position.

EXAMPLES OF ACTIVITIES

1. An activity performed in the upright 'stick' position and requiring head control can be developed in the following manner.

Primary activity
Purpose: head control.
Appreciation: water has weight.
Formation: a circle is formed, swimmer and therapist alternately, all holding hands and facing inwards.
Instruction: walk round sideways taking a step and bringing the other foot to it, lean and push against the water, when the water comes near your face—blow.

The points to watch are that the head is inclined in the direction the circle is moving and that it is maintained in such a position that the feet remain in contact with the floor of the bath and do not rise forwards or backwards and that the feet do not cross.

Follow-up activity
The purpose and formation remain the same, but appreciation is

increased in that when the swimmer feels the weight of water moving against him, he must push.

Instruction: walk sideways, clockwise; when the word 'change' is given, alter direction to anticlockwise.

Once the circle is moving well and the water is turbulent, the direction 'change' is given to ensure that the swimmer works with his head and trunk to move in the reverse direction.

Oblique activity

The purpose, appreciation and formation are the same again.

Instruction: walk round sideways stepping in the rhythm of a song or rhyme. For example, 'There was a crooked man who walked a crooked mile' or 'I'm forever blowing bubbles' for adults. The singing must continue and the rhythm be maintained when the direction is changed.

The point to watch here is that head control is subconsciously exerted and the swimmer is given plenty to remember to ensure that the reaction is automatic.

2. An activity using the 'ball' position.

Primary activity

Purpose: head control and body balance.

Appreciation: effect of the movement of the head on the body position in the water.

Formation: a circle is formed, alternately swimmer and therapist holding hands and facing inwards.

Instruction: swimmers bend your knees up towards your chests and slowly move your heads forwards and backwards.

Assistance is given to the swimmers by the therapists moving their arms forwards and backwards slightly. It is important that the head control forwards and backwards is such that the 'balled up' body does not swing too far.

Follow-up activity

Purpose: appreciation and formation remain the same.

Instruction: add to the previous instruction to sing a song—for example, Frère Jacques—and swing to its rhythm.

It is important to watch for automatic control by the head of the body swing and that 'blowing' occurs when the face is near the water on the forward movement.

Oblique activity
This follows the pattern of the above but can be progressed so that the body is gradually unrolled, a larger swing occurring but the head still controlling the body so that no sudden upthrust of the legs occurs.

3. This activity involves the 'ball' and 'stick' movement between the two postures.

Primary activity
Purpose: forward recovery.
Appreciation: extremes of posture; the effect of the head movement on the body position in the water.
Formation: swimmers are supported at the waist from behind by the therapists, all facing into a circle.
Instruction: sit in your chair, hands forward on the table, head back slowly until you are lying with your head on a shoulder.

When the word is given each swimmer bends his knees towards his chest, brings his head and hands forwards to reach for an object, blows and stands. Assistance is given to this forward movement. The points to watch are that the swimmer gets into the 'ball' shape, pushes forward with his head and hands, blows and balances in the erect position. Obtaining an object floating on the water, or reaching the bar, is important to the swimmer.

Follow-up activity
The purpose, appreciation, formation and instruction remain the same, but the swimmer is given less assistance to make the recovery off the therapist's hands.

Oblique activity
The purpose, appreciation, formation and instruction remain the same but no assistance is given and the activity may be made competitive by gradually reducing the number of objects.

UNDERWATER ACTIVITY
With the use of objects that will sink slowly the swimmer can begin to reach for them close to the surface, blowing when the water is near his face and gradually going deeper and deeper. He will have to keep his eyes open to see the object, important in all underwater activity, and also learn good breathing control and how to work down against the buoyancy of the water.

Further Reading

Association of Swimming Therapy for the Disabled (1981) EP Publishing.

Bolton, E. and Goodwin, D. (1974) *An Introduction to Pool Exercises*, 4th ed. Churchill Livingstone.

Guttman, L. (1973) Clinical aspects of spinal cord injuries. In: *Spinal Cord Injuries*, pp. 556–563. Blackwell Scientific.

Hyde, S. A. (1980) *Physiotherapy in Rheumatology*, Chap. 5. Blackwell Scientific.

Newman, J. (1975) *Swimming for Children with Physical and Sensory Impairments: Methods and Techniques for Therapy and Recreation.* Springfield, Illinois: Charles C. Thomas.

Reid, M. J. (1976) *Handling the Disabled Child in Water,* Association of Paediatric Chartered Physiotherapists.

Journal articles

Physiotherapy Vol. 57, No. 10 (1971):

Bickle, R. J.: Swimming pool management.

Bolton, E.: A technique of resistive exercise adapted for a small pool.

Cadogan, D. R.: Handling the handicapped.

Davis, B. C.: A technique of resistive exercise in the treatment pool.

Elkington, H. J.: The effective use of the pool.

Harris, S. J.: Bathside management, pool hygiene and resuscitation.

Trussell, E. C.: Swimming for the disabled.

Physiotherapy Vol. 64, No. 11 (1978):

Cadogan D. R.: Swimming: a physiotherapist's view.

Honnor A. T.: Swimming: the practicalities.

Physiotherapy Vol. 66, No. 2 (1980):

Harrison, R. A.: A quantitative approach to strengthening exercises in the hydrotherapy pool.

Leppard, B. J.: Tinea pedis.

Physiotherapy Vol. 67, No. 9 (1981):

Atkinson, G. P. and Harrison, R. A.: Implications of the Health and Safety at Work Act in relation to hydrotherapy departments.

Boyle, A. M.: The Bad Ragaz ring method.

Golland, A.: Basic hydrotherapy.

Physiotherapy Vol. 67, No. 10 (1981):

Harrison, R. A.: Tolerance of pool therapy by ankylosing spondylitis patients with low vital capacities.

Grasty, P. M.: Establishing a swimming club for disabled people.

Marten, J.: The Halliwick method.

Physiotherapy Vol. 68, No. 10 (1982):

Harrison, R. A. and Allard, L. L.: An attempt to quantify the resistance produced using the Bad Ragaz ring method.

Index